FITNESS ON THE BALL

A Core Program for Brain and Body

Anne Spalding

Crest View Elementary School

Linda E. Kelly, EdD

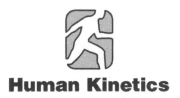

Human Kinetics

Library of Congress Cataloging-in-Publication Data

Spalding, Anne.
  Fitness on the ball : a core program for brain and body / Anne Spalding and Linda E. Kelly.
    p. cm.
  Includes bibliographical references.
  ISBN-13: 978-0-7360-6847-5 (soft cover)
  ISBN-10: 0-7360-6847-3 (soft cover)
1. Swiss exercise balls. 2. Exercise. I. Kelly, Linda E. II. Title.
  GV484.S63 2010
  613.7'10284--dc22

                          2009021778

ISBN: 978-0-7360-6847-5

Acquisitions Editor: Scott Wikgren; **Developmental Editor:** Amy Stahl; **Assistant Editors:** Lauren B. Morenz and Rachel Brito; **Copyeditor:** Patricia L. MacDonald; **Permission Manager:** Dalene Reeder; **Graphic Designer:** Joe Buck; **Graphic Artist:** Patrick Sandberg; **Cover Designer:** Keith Blomberg; **Photographer (cover):** Neil Bernstein; **Photographer (interior):** Neil Bernstein, except where otherwise noted. Photos on pp.19, 143, 167, 185, 192, 193, 194, and 227 © Anne Spalding; **Photo Asset Manager:** Laura Fitch; **Visual Production Assistant:** Joyce Brumfield; **Photo Production Manager:** Jason Allen; **Art Manager:** Kelly Hendren; **Associate Art Manager:** Alan L. Wilborn; **Illustrator:** Dragonfly Media Group and Mic Greenberg (illustrations on pp.14 and 15); **Printer:** Total Printing Systems

We thank Crest View Elementary School in Boulder, Colorado, for assistance in providing the location for the photo shoot for this book.

Printed in the United States of America   10 9 8 7 6 5 4 3

The paper in this book is certified under a sustainable forestry program.

Human Kinetics
Web site: www.HumanKinetics.com

United States: Human Kinetics
P.O. Box 5076
Champaign, IL 61825-5076
800-747-4457
e-mail: info@hkusa.com

Canada: Human Kinetics
475 Devonshire Road Unit 100
Windsor, ON N8Y 2L5
800-465-7301 (in Canada only)
e-mail: info@hkcanada.com

Europe: Human Kinetics
107 Bradford Road
Stanningley
Leeds LS28 6AT, United Kingdom
+44 (0) 113 255 5665
e-mail: hk@hkeurope.com

Australia: Human Kinetics
57A Price Avenue
Lower Mitcham, South Australia 5062
08 8372 0999
e-mail: info@hkaustralia.com

New Zealand: Human Kinetics
P.O. Box 80
Mitcham Shopping Centre, South Australia 5062
0800 222 062
e-mail: info@hknewzealand.com

E4052

Contents

Exercise Finder

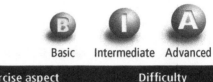

Basic Intermediate Advanced

Activity name	Page number	Exercise aspect	Difficulty
Chapter 5: Basic Positions			
Prone Position (Belly on the Ball)	39	Balance	B
Seated on the Ball (Bottom on the Ball)	41	Balance	B
Side on the Ball	43	Balance	B
Tabletop (Back on the Ball)	44	Balance	B
Chapter 6: Core Strength Exercises			
Dead Bug	49	Core strength	B
Novice Rainbow	50	Core strength	B
Back Extensions	51	Core strength	B
Spinal Twist for Strength	52	Core strength	B
Forward and Back	53	Core flexibility	B
Side to Side	54	Core flexibility	B
Hula	55	Core flexibility	B
Shoulder Shrug	55	Core flexibility	B
Seated Trunk Twist	56	Core flexibility	B
Torso Turners	58	Core strength	I

Preface

Welcome to *Fitness on the Ball*. You are about to dive into a book that explores the fascinating world of brain research and its relationship to fitness. You'll discover how using versatile and inexpensive equipment can improve your emotional state and sense of well-being. Exercise balls have become an integral part of the fitness industry, and their use has evolved over time. Exercise balls are used in a variety of ways and in a variety of settings.

Throughout our careers, Linda and I have been using exercise balls in our physical education classes and helping classroom teachers integrate balls into their curriculum. We've also been using the balls in our personal lives. Based on knowledge, research, and best practices, we know that incorporating the exercise ball or an active seating device into your life can contribute to your emotional and physical fitness. The following are experts and practitioners who have made significant contributions to our way of thinking, writing, teaching, and being:

- Classroom teachers
- SIED (significant identifiable emotional disability) teachers
- Special education teachers
- Physical education teachers
- Music and art teachers
- Literacy teachers
- Occupational and physical therapists
- Scientists
- Authors
- Pilates, Feldenkrais, and yoga instructors
- Personal trainers

Fitness on the Ball is for everyone—from babies to seniors. It highlights brain research as it relates to movement, emotions, and developments in fitness. It's different from *Kids on the Ball,* which we wrote with our friends Joanne Posner-Mayer and Janet Santopietro. The audience for that book is physical educators, occupational therapists, physical therapists, and all teachers working with kids. We know from talking to our readers that the audience for *Kids on the Ball* expanded to parents and the general public.

Fitness on the Ball explores specific uses, ideas, and concepts related to exercise balls, active seating devices, and something that may be new to you—sensory baskets. This book updates information in *Kids on the Ball* and explores the new areas mentioned earlier. It features new material and exercises written by Linda Kelly and me (Anne), two of the authors of *Kids on the Ball.* Our goal is to provide a user-friendly resource on using exercise balls, active seating devices, and sensory baskets that contribute to emotional and physical fitness. It also guides you toward a healthier, more balanced lifestyle.

Exercise balls have been gaining popularity over the years for a very good reason. They are fun, and fun motivates people to move. We've included information and advice on active seating devices, such as disks and wedges, because they are another safe and less obtrusive way to add movement in some otherwise sedentary-inducing spaces and places. They can improve posture, increase movement, and open airways for better breathing when used mindfully and with the guidance provided in this book. Active seating devices can be placed on chairs or stools, or they can replace traditional chairs.

The concept of adding movement throughout your day and not just before or after work or school is very deliberate. After reading *The Chair: Rethinking Culture, Body, and Design* by Galen Cranz, I had to dive a little deeper and expound on the use of exercise balls and active seating devices. Knowing that the movement toward alternative seating was gaining momentum in the areas of sociology and architecture was both inspiring and motivating. We realized these concepts could be more universally accepted and even embraced. We hope you'll pick up some fun, healthy habits that will activate your lifestyle.

Inactivity is a health hazard and is a leading cause of death in the United States. There's also an issue with some of us type As being on the run all the time. In this book you'll see the phrase *regulate your way through the day*. This means all of us forming new habits of interspersing activity with relaxation.

This book offers you some tools to make modifications to your daily life. Vigorous activities followed by calming activities can bring balance to a hectic day and increase productivity. You'll feel a sense of physical and emotional stability when you start to treat yourself to a little more movement with a sense of playfulness.

An additional component of this book is the concept of sensory baskets. These baskets, boxes, or bags contain items that both calm and stimulate your senses. Think about your senses right now: seeing, smelling, hearing, feeling, and touching. Being more aware of your senses is vital when you try to maintain balance and productivity throughout the day. In the later chapters of this book, we give you suggestions about organizing items that will help you balance your senses. We take an existing idea and suggest its use in places other than the occupational therapy, physical therapy, and hospice communities where we found them. We want to take sensory integration into the mainstream.

I got so excited about all these balance concepts that I started my own Web site: www.anneontheball.com. I couldn't capture all of my ideas and fit them into this book, so the overflow will go on the Web site. You can go there to see and hear ideas for people of all ages who are trying to find or maintain balance in their lives. The Web site will grow over time and include the following:

- Essays, photos, and ideas from me (Anne) and various readers of this book
- Products we love and recommend
- Connections and links to related topics
- Activity sheets to help you focus on proper mechanics and account for sets of exercises completed

I hope www.anneontheball.com will be a site you'll visit often and that we'll all develop together.

Acknowledgments

I want to acknowledge and thank my coauthor, Linda Kelly, for her patience, time, and commitment. Her expertise was invaluable. This book has been more of a personal journey than I ever would have anticipated. Bringing together the emotional, social, and physical dimensions of daily exercise was a lofty goal, and I hope we've achieved it.

My long-time mentor and friend, Anne Turnacliff, was a guardian angel to me while I was stressing out over how to weave personal stories into this text. Anne has the patience of a saint and knew I wouldn't be happy until the ball went over the net, so to speak. Her hours spent helping me edit are priceless, as is her friendship.

My friends, co-workers, students, and family are the foundation of my life, and I want to thank all of you for hanging in there with me. You inspired and motivated me to pursue my passion—to teach and write in the educational field.

Here's to a brighter and lighter future now that one more thing is off my list and the ball is in your hands.

Love and best wishes.

Anne

I am grateful to my co-author, Anne Spalding, for her steadfast focus on this project in the midst of teaching full-time, learning Spanish to connect with her students, taking care of her parents, and trying to have a life and maintain her sanity. We met and worked at her home, shared the trials of writing and rewriting (and rewriting) along with good snacks, lots of frustration, and laughter. Anne is quite a woman, colleague, and friend.

I thank my husband, Jim Rhoads, for being on his own during the Saturdays (and occasional Sundays) plus the many school holidays that Anne and I spent working. You are truly a loving and caring person and husband. You even helped during the photo shoot! Thanks for taking that burden.

I am indebted to my children, Michael and Elizabeth, for giving their time for our preliminary photo shoot. You gave us great templates to show the models at the shoot. And Lizzy, thanks for batting clean-up. Michael, I missed you at the shoot; however, you had to keep your commitment.

Anne Turnacliff assisted us in ways too numerous to list. Thanks for all the writing and editing you did, along with moral and physical support. You really deserve third-author credit. Wayne Turnacliff, thanks to you also. You were a critical stagehand.

Scott Wikgren, Amy Stahl, Rachel Brito, and the other folks at HK, whom we may never know, thanks! You worked hard on our behalf. We do appreciate it.

Linda Kelly

MODELS ACKNOWLEDGMENTS

Models, where can we begin! Thanks for taking the time to be with us at the photo shoot. You were patient, serious, funny, and delightful. You gave us your best effort and we know you will love your photos as much as we do! You are the best!

Nicki Bailey
Fielden Batey
Marc Bekoff
Bev Buchler
Melissa Capparo
Donna Casey
Jonny Coletta
Rohini Dasan
Alan Sangabriel Davila
Andy L. Carcia Davila
Jannal Garcia Davila
Marcela Davila
Milton Sangabriel Davila
Raquel Davila
Teresa Davila
Benjamin Davis
Christopher Davis
Isabelle Davis
Harriet Edelstein
Jeri Eurich
Sarah Filley
Marilyn Fogerty
Kelly R. Garza
Veronica Gebremariam
Monique Guidry
Tracy Halgren
Cassie Hickman
Aiden Houck
Joshua Houck
Becky Houghton
Jill Johnson
Ellie Marie Jones
Kathleen Jones

Patrick Jones
Connor Kellermyer
Zoe Kellermyer
Nancy Kissinger
Paula Kissinger
Ewan Robert Lester
Audrey Leonard
Donna Mason
Cade Mead
Emma Mead
Tatum Mead
Zoe Movshovitz
Kevin Rauhauser
William Redding
Nicole Reno
Rick Reynolds
Elizabeth Rhoads
Jim Rhoads
Angie J. Rioddleberger
Chelsea Rowan
Malia Sharp
Frieda Silva
Marco Silva
Al Spalding
Mary Spalding
Henry Stone
Ivy Stone
Laura Stone
Kenneth Suslak
Anne Turnacliff
Wayne Turnacliff
Clarke Yeager

How to Use the CD-ROM

The bound-in CD-ROM allows you to copy and paste any of the illustrations and exercise photos from this book. You can use the images in slides for a PowerPoint presentation or in traditional overheads, posters, notes, handheld visuals, and assessments. Be sure to get out the CD-ROM, load it on your computer, and explore all that it has to offer. It includes a glossary of terms that you can print and post. Visual aids, printouts, and posters contain reminders and cues on using the ball and exercises. Assessment forms allow you to customize exercises for yourself or for your patients or clients and ensure proper technique.

Because of the popularity of the activities and lesson plans in our original book, *Kids on the Ball*, we've included them on the CD-ROM as well. You'll find 118 activities and 23 complete lesson plans that have been successfully used by teachers in physical education classes to help children develop balance, coordination, rhythm, and fitness skills.

Want to modify your lifestyle? Could you use a little more balance in your life? Need some strategies and ideas to make the change? Often change is simpler to achieve than believed. Exercising on the ball, modifying your seating, and using sensory baskets are easy, fun ways to optimize your fitness and well-being. This new lifestyle is at your fingertips. So keep reading—and moving. Here's to your future. We think it's going to be brighter now that you're getting on the ball.

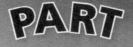
Exercise Balls and Active Seating Devices: From Benefits to Assessments

In part I you'll find everything you need to get on the ball. Chapter 1 covers the benefits and reasons for using exercise balls and active seating devices. Chapter 2 discusses the specifics of selecting exercise balls and safety considerations. Chapter 3 addresses storage and management of the balls. New storage choices have become available since we wrote *Kids on the Ball* in 1999, so be sure to check out chapter 3 even if you have read *Kids on the Ball*. Assessment suggestions and ideas, proper mechanics, and posture are all included in chapter 4. The addition of the book's bound-in CD-ROM has made the customized options for assessment and record keeping more efficient and effective. Chapter 4 also addresses social and emotional challenges as they relate to learning experiences and exercise. We think you'll find this information helpful while working with the exercise ball on your own or with friends, family, and groups.

one

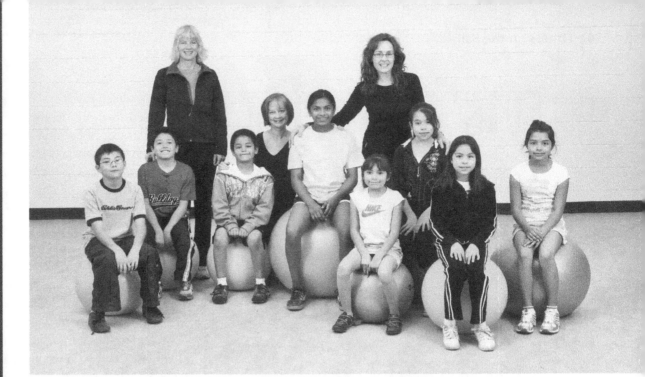

Benefits of Using Exercise Balls

E xercise balls provide immediate and dramatic feedback to the user. When a person sits or exercises on this unstable piece of equipment in a safe manner, things happen fast. Your central nervous system wakes up, like an alarm clock going off in the morning. It puts you in a more alert state. The change from a hard chair to an exercise ball is energizing.

This inexpensive and multiuse piece of exercise equipment can be referred to as an **exercise ball**, stability ball, FitBall, physio ball, and Swiss ball. Over time a wide variety of adaptations have been made while keeping the benefits of the exercise ball in mind. The FitBall is available with feet so that it stays in place, and that makes it a good choice for use as a chair at home, work, schools, clinics, and fitness centers. There is also a FitBall Peanut designed for beginners, people with special needs, or people recovering from injuries. The newest fitness and sensory tool is a smaller, donut-shaped exercise ball that would also fit into a variety of settings to use for exercise and alternative seating. The FitBall Donut and Peanut offer comfortable and secure choices for training and seating for everyone from children to seniors (see figure 1.1).

More active seating options that we find helpful in ordinarily sedentary settings are as follows:

- FitBall Seating Discs
- FitBall Wedges
- FitBall Air Cushions
- Movin'Sit Air Cushions

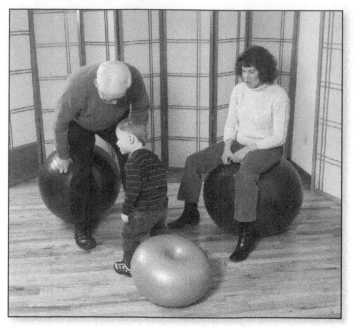

Figure 1.1 Alternative seating for infants to seniors, including the FitBall donut.

All these alternatives and options are discussed in more detail in chapter 13 on classroom use and chapter 14 on home and work use. They add wonderful choices to increase movement throughout the day.

Sitting, rocking, rolling, and stretching on an exercise ball stimulate the central nervous system while also increasing blood flow and maximizing brain functioning. An abundance of brain research confirms that movement wakes up the brain and makes it more efficient and effective. So why do we keep asking people to sit down, be quiet, and get some work done for long periods of time? Probably because we have the mistaken notion that one must sit quietly to be productive. In his book *The Learning Brain*, Eric Jensen (1995) includes an amazing number of facts about the physiology and biology of the brain. Following is one of the many interesting facts quoted from Jensen's book:

> *Research summary: Many learners are asked to remain in their seats and to remain quiet for optimal learning. But research by Della Valle et al. in 1984 says that may not be a good idea. Among adolescents, 50% of the learners needed "extensive mobility while learning." Of the remaining 50% half of those (25%) needed occasional mobility and the remaining needed minimal movement opportunities. (p. 114)*

This research finding is just one example of how to look at the range of movement required by different people to stay focused. People have different styles of thinking, working, learning, and doing things. If we are in search of ways to be more efficient and effective at what we do, then using a ball as a chair and exercising on it may help. Using an exercise ball has been shown to affect educational and work settings for a variety of people who may not function to their maximum capacity when the setting does not have alternatives to traditional chairs. In his article "Active Classroom Frees Kids From Desk Chairs" (2006), classroom teacher Phil Rynearson encourages his students to use exercise balls to improve focus and burn calories. This is an innovative approach from Dr. James Levine, a Mayo Clinic researcher, who promotes more movement for deskbound workers and students alike. Top all that off with the fact that exercise balls are relatively inexpensive, and we think you'll be wanting to add an exercise ball or two to your life.

The concept of changing our state of alertness offers an opportunity for improved productivity, increased fitness, and playful fun in public and private facilities. Most of us appreciate a regularly scheduled break. Using the exercise ball and other alternative seating options can give your brain and body a break. These options also have the potential to relieve stress, discomfort, and the monotony of some tasks.

In the remainder of the chapter, we will discuss balance, our ability to remain upright, and how to avoid falls in a variety of settings. Balance is a skill that we need so we avoid getting hurt and it contributes to our motor performance. We test it every day when we stand and move around. Using the balls and active seating devices strengthens and trains our cores while improving our sense of balance. Improving balance while using this equipment is *fun*! Most of us tend to do things that have a *fun factor*, and exercise balls and alternative seating options have a fun factor that we think you'll enjoy. In addition to having fun, they offer a lot of versatility and contribute to the development of functional fitness. Educational benefits that are derived from being engaged in more active learning environments are being validated through ongoing brain research and books that are cited in this book. The relatively low cost of modifying our daily environments with the addition of active seating and exercise options at work and home add up to make this a must-read chapter.

BALANCE

Our need to perceive movement and space is what keeps us from falling in our daily lives, and it is important in preventing injuries throughout our lives. Each time we interact with an exercise ball, our brains and bodies are alerted to the movements, large or small, that occur. The lack of stability in an exercise ball is key to improving **balance**, which is the ability to resist gravity and remain upright and steady.

In the book *The Brain That Changes Itself: Stories of Personal Triumph From the Frontiers of Brain Science*, Norman Doidge, MD, discusses what he calls a "neuroplastic revolution." Doidge gives vivid examples of people of all ages with a wide variety of neurological conditions undergoing amazing transformations that until now were unheard of. One example he uses to discuss posture is from Pascual-Leone, where they compare sled riding down a hill and making "tracks" to the neural pathways in the brain. "If we develop poor posture, it becomes hard to correct. If we develop good habits, they too become solidified" (Doidge 2007, pp. 208-209).

Making postural adjustments on the ball when a person starts to lose his balance is an example of allowing a person to test and practice the balance reflex that he needs in a safe setting. We've watched young children through senior citizens practice balancing on the ball and have seen the improvement in their posture and core strength. We also believe in combination with other educational practices that the ability to recover from a loss of balance is improved.

FUN

Everyone may not comprehend the brain benefits of using an exercise ball or alternative seating option when they first try out ideas listed in this book. They'll probably just like using exercise balls and alternative seating options because they are fun. So, what better way to entice everyone to be physically active? The sizes and colors of exercise balls and alternative seating options are so alluring that very few individuals are not attracted to one or more of them. If fun encourages people, young and old, to use exercise balls and alternative seating options, that is a huge benefit. In our increasingly sedentary society, physical activity must be promoted at every opportunity in fun and playful ways. For our purposes in this book, **physical activity** is moving the body, and it includes house and yard work as well as sport and fitness activities.

VERSATILITY

An unlimited number of exercises can be performed on the ball. **Pilates**, **yoga**, **Feldenkrais**, and other movement systems and exercises have all been integrated into ball exercises, expanding the number of activities that can be done with this one piece of equipment. Few other pieces of equipment, if any, can make that claim. Exercise balls are very versatile, and they can develop four fitness components: strength, flexibility, balance, and cardiorespiratory fitness. In part II of this book you will find exercises to help develop all four of these fitness areas. We've made sure you have photos of all the exercises, both in the chapters and on the bound-in CD-ROM, so you can make good use of them.

FUNCTIONAL FITNESS

Using an exercise ball promotes **functional fitness**, or the fitness necessary to perform daily functions. It is the perfect piece of equipment to improve **core strength**, which is the strength of the muscles in the **torso**, especially the smaller intrinsic ones, and is the basis for all movement and literally the core of our daily life. The body's core consists of all the muscles in the torso, from the small deep muscles in the pelvis, back, chest, and abdominal area to the more well-known larger muscles of the body (**abdominal muscles**, **trapezius**, **pectoralis major**, and **latissimus dorsi**). A weak core can result in a back injury, while a strong core improves posture and helps maintain balance and performance when participating in physical activity or enjoying a sport.

In *O, the Oprah Magazine* (February 2009), an article on posture power emphasizes the importance of posture in a workout. The article states, "In a review of more than 100 studies, scientists from UCLA found that poor posture is associated with breathing problems, falls, depression, and decreased quality of life, all of which shave years off of life expectancy" (p. 197). We think the exercise ball is an indispensable tool for achieving proper alignment and posture for people of all ages in many settings.

EDUCATION

In addition to the physical and health benefits, there are education benefits associated with using exercise balls. For now, we'll focus on the connection between physical and emotional states and use of the exercise ball. Later, in chapter 13, you can read more about using exercise balls in various classroom settings to improve focus and productivity. Finally, in chapter 14, we address the workplace environments of people of all ages who are dealing with attention issues.

In our combined experience of more than 50 years of teaching, we have seen improvement in concentration while people use the exercise ball and alternative seating options. Sitting and bouncing on the exercise ball can promote a calm state. Fidgeting can be reduced by gentle bouncing on an exercise ball or a shifting of body weight while using an alternative seating option. We've seen the "distractor factor" issue virtually eliminated.

Alternative seating options have been noted for improving alertness as well as promoting a calm state. The alertness is derived from the increased blood flow through the brain, spine, and back. When people are seated on an exercise ball, wedge, or disc, they frequently adjust their posture, and this allows for chest expansion and increases lung capacity.

A recent publication by John J. Ratey (2008), "Spark: The Revolutionary New Science of Exercise and the Brain," dives into a favorite topic—the connection between exercise and the brain. Ratey states, "Even there, in the roots of our biology, they've found signs of the body's influence on the mind. It turns out that moving our muscles produces proteins that travel through the bloodstream and into the brain, where they play pivotal roles in the mechanics of our highest thought processes" (p. 5). On the back of the same book there is a quote from Greg LeMond, three-time winner of the Tour de France that states, "This book is a real turning point that explains something I've been trying to figure out for years, having experienced symptoms of both ADHD and mild depression. Exercise is not simply necessary; it's medicine."

At the end of my last school year, I (Anne) had a parent who came in and wanted to know why, after all the consultations she had with experts and specialists, I seemed to be the one person who really understood her child. Why had I been able to understand what her child was going through and seemed to need? I felt pressure to explain myself. It was a tipping-point moment for me. I had to tell her I knew because I had experienced similar situations myself. I have symptoms of ADD (attention-deficit disorder), and so I understand it from a very personal perspective. At age three I lost my left eye and have very successfully navigated my way through life thus far with the use of only one eye. Combining a vision loss at a very young age with ADD has created a unique way of seeing and feeling the world. I have received awards for my teaching and have written and spoken publicly throughout my career. I am constantly using strategies and modifications to be efficient and effective as a teacher, coworker, and friend. The exercise ball has proven to be important to me in finding my balance in life.

ADD/ADHD, autism, and all special needs are very specific to each person. There is no one-size-fits-all answer to any of it. All these disorders have a spectrum from mild to severe. Some experts say that there are characteristics related to sensory integration challenges and distractibility issues experienced by all of us at different times. The way that every person and family manages and copes with these special needs varies greatly. With professional guidance, education, and lots of patience, people dealing with all of these conditions can hopefully find peace, happiness, and productivity.

At one point in my career I had a student in class whose autism was very severe. He always had a paraprofessional come with him to physical education class. One day I was working with him and his class using the exercise balls. I happened to be playing some African drum music on this particular day. I will never forget looking over and seeing him directly in front of the stereo speaker, bouncing on the ball to the drum beat and looking happier and calmer than I had ever seen him before. I felt incredibly joyful that this boy finally looked calm and content after seeing him in many different autistic states, including head banging.

In 2006, I attended a Brain Basics Convention hosted by Kim Bevill, founder of Gray Matters, which brings together the latest brain research and education. At this conference I had the opportunity to hear one of my favorite authors, Eric Jensen, speak about the seven neurological breakthroughs. In his book *Learning Smarter: The New Science of Teaching*, Jensen (2000, p. 173) cites a study by Ericksson and colleagues (1998) wherein they note that "the hippocampus, the area of the brain linked to learning and memory, retains its ability to generate neurons throughout life, even into old age." In his action steps in the same book, Jensen repeatedly suggests exposing learners to enriched learning experiences, including physical activity.

LOW COST

Last, but certainly not least in the list of benefits of using exercise balls, is the low cost. Exercise balls are relatively inexpensive, especially when compared with the purchase of other exercise equipment, chairs, and stools. Purchasing exercise balls is a good investment. At a cost ranging at the present time between $20+ for a small child-sized ball to $30+ for a larger adult-sized ball, an exercise ball provides high utility for minimal cost. We list our top recommendations for where to purchase quality exercise balls in the resources section in the back of this book.

SUMMARY

Exercise balls can help improve balance, functional fitness, and many people's abilities to focus and get more work accomplished. Exercise balls challenge us both physically and emotionally to be effective and efficient at work and at home. They are relatively inexpensive, versatile, and fun to use.

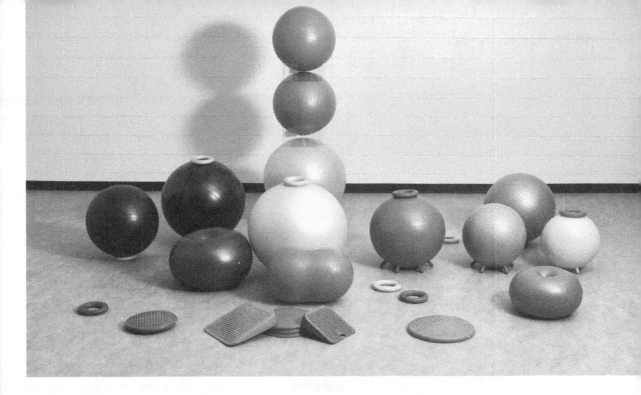

Selection and Safety of Exercise Balls

A n exercise ball program must be safe to be effective and fun. To provide this safe environment, it's essential to become knowledgeable about ball sizing, instructions for inflating the exercise ball, safety considerations, and proper use of the ball. This chapter covers these topics, which are critical for integrating balls into any setting.

SELECTING THE CORRECT EXERCISE BALL SIZE

Selecting an exercise ball is based on height, body proportion, and weight. Figure 2.1 shows the exercise ball user seated in the correct posture for measuring the ball size. The crucial variable when selecting the correct ball size is the angle at the knees formed by the hips, knees, and feet. The angle should be 90 degrees or slightly greater. This angle provides the optimal body position for good posture. Because people of the same height have different leg lengths and different torso lengths, a slight adjustment in size (by letting air out, by adding air, or by choosing a larger ball) may be necessary.

Exercise balls come in a variety of colors and styles, now including balls with little feet that look a bit like cow udders, such as FitBall with feet and Pezzi Sitsolution Maxafe, both of which are available in burst-resistant and original material (see figure 2.2). With or without the little feet, a burst-resistant exercise ball helps protect against rapid deflation should the ball be punctured. Buying a ball that goes with your home or office decor has the added dimension of blending into the surrounding space. Check the resources section in the back of this book for our recommendation of a supplier that offers the latest related items, available in a variety of sizes and colors. Most balls

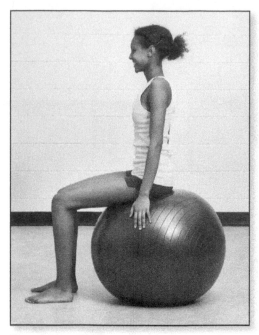

Figure 2.1 Sitting on the ball correctly.

we've used are marked with centimeters or inches on the ball and on the box so you can measure them and fill them up accordingly. *Note:* The size marked refers to the *maximum* inflation size. Never overinflate an exercise ball. Like a balloon, the polyvinyl will thin out as it expands and be prone to puncture. Under-inflation is preferred and is more comfortable for the user.

PROPERLY FITTING THE EXERCISE BALL TO THE USER

If you are selecting an exercise ball for use in your home or office, you will want to pick the color you like and the size using the following height chart as a guide. The measurements in the chart are the circumference of the ball when inflated to its maximum size. If you are at the upper end of the height scale and a little heavier, you might want to go up a size. It is softer and more comfortable for some people to have a larger, slightly underinflated ball.

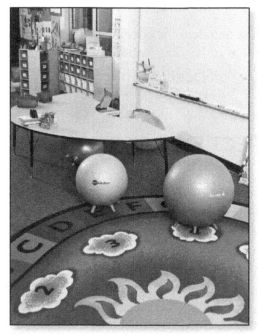

Figure 2.2 Exercise ball with feet.

Age and Height Measurements

5 years to 4'8" (142 cm)	45 cm
4'8" to 5'3" (142 cm to 160 cm)	55 cm
5'3" to 6'0" (160 cm to 183 cm)	65 cm
6'0" to 6'7" (183 cm to 201 cm)	75 cm

When buying for a medical practice, health club, or school, you can use the previous chart as a guide and assess the size and weight of your users. The comfort and safety of the person using the ball is important, and a ball that is slightly larger than the 90-degree angle of the knees is acceptable, but it is not recommended to use a ball that is too small. When working on some stretches and balances, a ball that is too big will hinder success. In some educational settings, we've had people use one ball during upright bouncing-type exercises and then switch to a slightly smaller ball when working on balance and stretches.

INFLATING EXERCISE BALLS

Most exercise balls come packaged deflated with two plugs; one plug is a spare. Keep all spare plugs in a container because plugs are easily lost; do not throw away extra plugs. Before inflating, make sure the ball is at room temperature. You should use a compressor to inflate the exercise balls because they require a high volume of air at low pressure, which a compressor has. A bicycle pump will not work when inflating exercise balls because it delivers a low volume of air at high pressure.

Both electric air compressors and manual air raft or mattress pumps that have a cone-shaped nozzle will work. Car or tire repair facilities have compressors that they might be willing to let you use. Although gas stations have air compressors, the nozzle is not cone shaped and must have a valve stem to initiate the airflow.

I purchased the electric pump shown in figure 2.3 at a local hardware store. It is on wheels, has a compartment that holds a variety of attachments, and has been working well for inflating new balls.

The invention of a small handheld dual-action pump (often sold in the balloon section of equipment catalogs)—one brand is called the Faster Blaster—makes it possible to inflate a ball without a compressor. You will definitely want one, and at less than $10, maybe two. Sometimes balls are packaged with a ball pump. Although it is possible to fully inflate a ball with the hand pump, it takes time and effort. It is not the way to inflate an entire set of exercise balls for your group. It is,

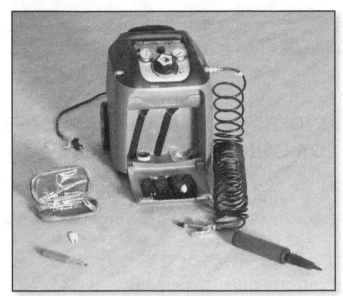

Figure 2.3 Electric pump on wheels.

however, essential for the little bit of air, or topping off, that balls sometimes need. The pump also allows you to inflate a ball a little more for a person who needs a slightly larger ball that has been previously deflated for another person in a previous group.

Figure 2.4 shows the correct way to measure a ball. It is best to check to see if the ball fits the person after it has been inflated to the desired size. In many instances this size will be comfortable, but we always have a plug puller to let air out. The size is marked on the ball and the box. Mark the desired height of the ball on a wall for initial inflation. Use a book or clipboard to make a 90-degree angle to see if the ball is in the appropriate range for maximum safety and comfort. This is accomplished by placing the clipboard on top of the legs while the person is seated to look for the 90-degree angle. Remember not to overinflate the exercise ball.

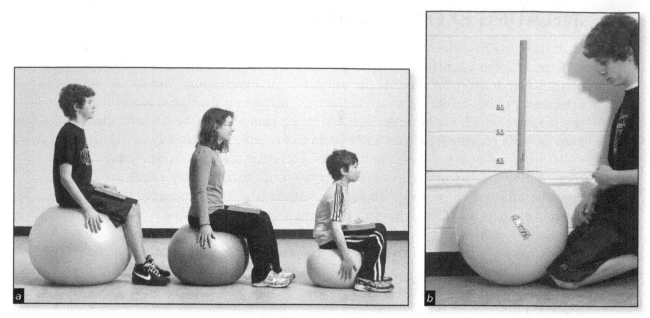

Figure 2.4 *(a)* Clipboard 90-degree angle check with measurements of 17 inches (43 cm), 21 inches (53 cm), or 25 inches (65 cm); *(b)* measurements marked on tape on the wall.

UNDERSTANDING GENERAL SAFETY GUIDELINES FOR USING EXERCISE BALLS

General safety guidelines while using an exercise ball should be considered in all settings. An exercise ball is not a toy, and it should be used only as a chair or a piece of equipment to exercise with and on. It should always be used with care and caution. Here are two lists of general safety guidelines, one for protecting the person using the ball and the other for protecting the ball.

Protecting the Participant

1. Wear any clothing that you feel comfortable wearing while seated on the ball or performing exercises.
2. Take caution when wearing belts, watches, or other sharp objects that could puncture the ball.
3. Always maintain optimal posture while seated on the ball. *Note:* Do not twist, bend, or rotate the spine while bouncing on the ball.
4. Follow instructions to maximize your results while exercising on the ball. Overexuberance can result in injuries.
5. Move slowly and mindfully when on an exercise ball.
6. Always be cautious about your head and neck alignment.
7. If you are teaching, stop your instruction if people are not in control of their movements. Safety should always come first.

Protecting the Ball

1. The floor should be clean and free of anything sharp, such as pins, staples, or other sharp items.
2. Carpet, wood, tartan, or other artificial floors are all surfaces where an exercise ball can be used safely.
3. The space where the exercise balls are used can vary depending on the desired use of the ball. In part II of the book, which includes exercises you can do on the exercise ball, we will show a small icon like this for exercises that are appropriate for small desk spaces. Other exercises will show an icon like this for exercises that need unobstructed space, with approximately three feet (1 m) around each participant's exercise ball.
4. Caution should be taken when a user is wearing belts, watches, or other sharp objects that could puncture the ball.
5. A person can sit on a ball with any type of footwear as long as the size of the ball looks correct with the shoes being worn.

small space

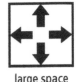

large space

Safety Training: Protecting the Brain and Spinal Cord

Lesson Objectives

At the end of this discussion or lesson, the user will be able to do the following:

1. Explain the importance of the brain and the spinal cord.
2. Tell how to prevent injury when exercising on the ball.

Vocabulary

- command center
- nervous system
- on balance
- off balance

Setting Up for Safety

1. Discuss back and head injuries with the users. Ask if anyone knows of someone who has had a serious neck or back injury or problem. (Christopher Reeve is a prominent and potent example. Younger students may need a more current example, if they do not know someone.)
2. Display a picture, poster, or model of the skeletal system. Reproduce and use figure 2.5 if needed.
3. Have users name and point to the bones they know.
4. Explain how the **brain** connects to the **spinal cord**, housed in the base of the **neck** and the back.
5. Have users touch their **heads**. Tell the users, *Under the hair and scalp and inside the **skull** is the brain, which is approximately the size of your two fists.*

6. Show students a poster of the **nervous system**, and point out the brain and spinal cord. Reproduce and use figure 2.6 if needed.

7. Explain: *The brain is the **command center** for all bodily functions, and messages travel up and down the spinal cord, connecting the brain with the rest of the body.* It is helpful to illustrate the concept by giving the students some examples of how the brain works. For example, tell students, *When we want to run, jump, or climb stairs, the brain sends the message down the spinal cord and then to the nerves of the muscles in the legs so movement will occur. When we reach for something that is hot and may burn us, the nerves in the hand send a message up the spinal cord to the brain, and the brain sends an immediate message back down the spinal cord and out to the nerves of the muscles in the hand, telling the hand to pull away.*

8. Finally, tell users, *The **vertebrae** and skull are the bony structures that protect our spinal cord and brain. If we are hit or fall hard, the vertebrae or skull may not withstand the impact.* Make it clear to the users that when the spinal cord or brain is damaged, messages can become weak or scrambled or may no longer be transmitted to and from the brain.

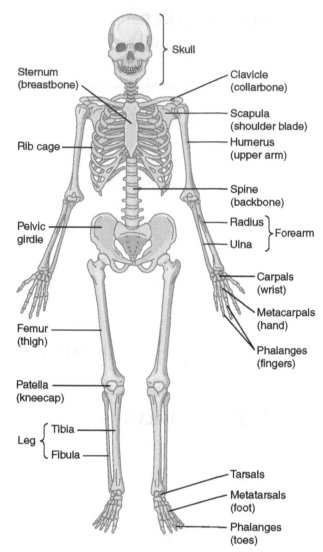

Figure 2.5 Skeletal system.

Reprinted, by permission, from M. Flegel, 2008, *Sport first aid*, 4th ed. (Champaign, IL: Human Kinetics), 32.

9. Assure users that knowing how their bodies work and following directions will help them prevent injuries. Emphasize: *Never do anything on the ball that might cause you to injure your vertebrae, skull, brain, or spinal cord.*

10. Review the terms **on balance** and **off balance** by asking the users the following questions: *Can you give a definition of on balance and off balance?* Answer: On balance is not falling. Off balance is falling.

    What should you do if you sense you are going off balance? Answer: Slow down or stop.

11. Explain to the users the following information about staying on balance (see figure 2.7). *You are the experts on what is happening to your body, and I know that each of you will exercise responsibly and with control. Occasionally while you are learning control, you might not recognize that you are close to being off balance, or*

out of control. However, do not worry, because I will let you know by asking you to get off the ball, sit on the floor, and observe me or others who are in control. There are many ways to learn. Hearing, seeing, and doing are my favorites. After you watch and listen, I'm sure you'll be ready to work safely on the ball.

SUMMARY

Follow the guidelines in this chapter for selecting, fitting, inflating, and using exercise balls to prevent injury and increase your understanding of how to keep yourself and others safe when using an exercise ball. Use the lesson provided in this chapter as a guide to exercise ball safety before bringing out this fun and exciting equipment within an educational, therapeutic, or fitness center setting. With proper care and precaution, your exercise balls will last, and you and your group will enjoy safe and productive exercise on the ball for a long time to come. Be sure to read chapter 3 to learn about storage ideas, distribution, and management of exercise balls.

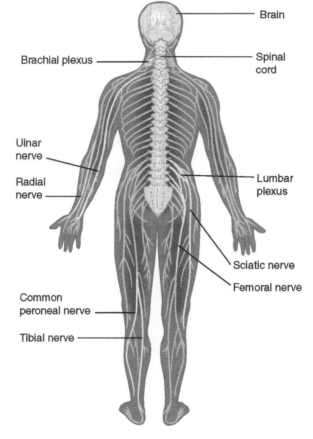

Figure 2.6 Nervous system.

Reprinted, by permission, from M. Flegel, 2008, *Sport first aid*, 4th ed. (Champaign, IL: Human Kinetics), 34.

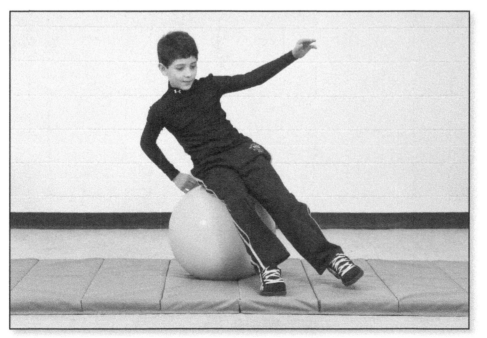

Figure 2.7 Starting to lose balance on the exercise ball.

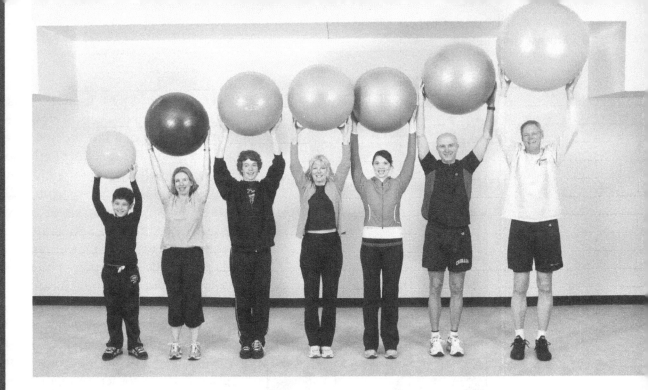

Storage, Distribution, and Management of Exercise Balls

• •

Adding exercise balls to your home, school, workplace, or care facility can be easy or a challenge. In your home, for example, it may be easy to set up a few safety guidelines, such as when, where, and how the exercise ball can be used. However, it may take additional organization and planning to use exercise balls in a school, care facility, or workplace. Using exercise balls in any environment is beneficial because the results are enthusiastic participants developing strong, flexible bodies. In this chapter we give you a variety of successful storage, distribution, and management strategies and techniques that you can adapt or adopt.

STORAGE

After *Kids on the Ball* was published, I (Anne) got my dream job at Crest View Elementary, a school very close to my home. I had a cage built to hold the exercise balls in the back of my main storage room (see figure 3.1), which worked well for starters.

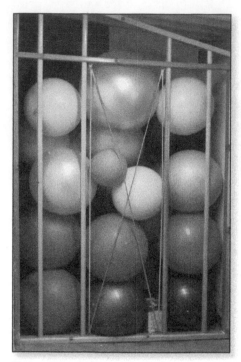

Figure 3.1 Ball cage built for storage of exercise balls.

Over the years, I have used the balls more and had classroom teachers borrow the balls for their rooms, too. It has become necessary to add a second ball cage closer to the door for the storage of balls that are used for physical education and classrooms (see figure 3.2). This allows for quicker, easier access to the exercise balls as we need them. I have found that the easier it is to access the balls, the more they are used. It's a bit like the popular phrase used in real estate: location, location, location.

Storage in an office or home setting can be handled in different ways. Balls with legs are available for easy use and storage. If you are using a ball without legs you can store it by placing it in a corner, propping it against another object, or stacking it on a clear ring. See figure 3.3 for other options for storing a ball. Purchasing details are found in the resources section of this book.

Wherever you are using the balls, remember to store them carefully and keep them away from direct heat sources and sharp objects. Be mindful of the fact that they are very alluring to anyone who passes by. It is best to post a sign near the balls with directions for sitting on them correctly (see printable, reproducible poster on CD-ROM) so that people will know they need to be careful. The balls are not toys. They are exercise equipment that comes with precautions like other exercise equipment.

DISTRIBUTION

As with other equipment, distributing exercise balls in an efficient and effective manner is a fine art. We revise our procedures according to each situation. Being specific when demonstrating exactly how you want everyone to handle the exercise balls and why you want them to handle the exercise balls with care will make all the difference in keeping the environment safe and productive. Adults and kids might be tempted to toss, throw, or bounce a ball with too much force when retrieving the balls. That is why we use caution and reminders about safety so that no one gets hurt and nothing gets broken.

We suggest the following tips when distributing the exercise balls:

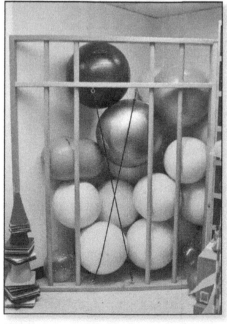

Figure 3.2 Second ball cage built at Anne's school for easier access for physical education and classroom teachers who borrow exercise balls.

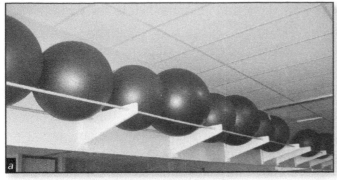

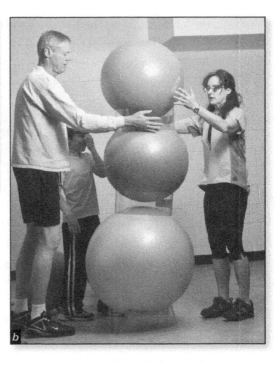

Figure 3.3 Other possible storage options: *(a)* horizontal shelving to hold balls off the ground and *(b)* clear stackable rings.

© Anne Spalding

- When working with large groups, always have several different locations for participants to retrieve balls.
- Create temporary ball bins to house the balls using cones, chairs, or benches.
- Send a few people at a time to retrieve the balls from an easy-access location.
- Demonstrate how the ball should be carried to the work space. It can be held with two hands at waist height or overhead (see figure 3.4).
- Define the exercise space by describing the amount of room that will be needed to extend arms and legs without touching or kicking others.
- Markers or spots can be used to designate safe locations to exercise.

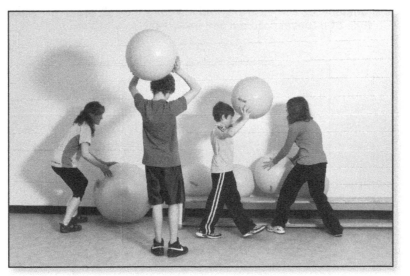

Figure 3.4 Students holding and carrying the balls at waist height and overhead.

- When putting the ball away, always walk, lean, and place the ball in the designated location (see figure 3.5*a*).
- A bucket brigade type of formation is effective and efficient when retrieving and putting away balls for large groups (see figure 3.5*b*).

A short, meaningful conversation with whomever you are working with to reinforce distribution procedures sets the foundation for management of the balls. It is a good idea to really drive the message home with a pair-and-share discussion. For example, *Please turn to your neighbor or a small group close to you and share between one and three things you need to keep in mind when getting out, using, and putting away the exercise balls.*

Most people love to talk, and giving them clear guidelines about what they are discussing makes the pair-and-share process quick, easy, and effective (see figure 3.6). Always let people know that you'll be listening in to be sure the safety guidelines "stuck" with them. People get used to this process and can do it quickly. When working with larger groups if you have time, you can ask groups to share their findings without repeating other groups' conclusions. See more details on the pair-and-share assessment strategy in chapter 4, "Assessment, Proper Mechanics, and Social and Emotional Challenges."

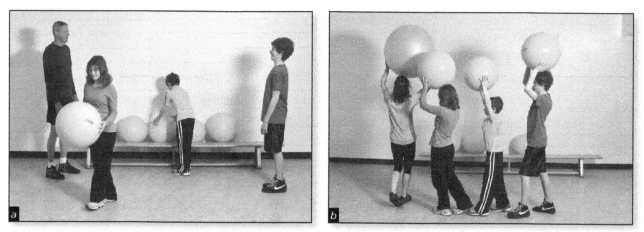

Figure 3.5 *(a)* Postural alignment used when lifting and lowering the ball, especially when putting the ball away; *(b)* bucket brigade style of retrieving and putting away balls.

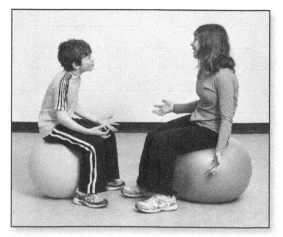

Figure 3.6 Group pairing and sharing while seated on balls.

MANAGEMENT: GYMNASIUMS, CLASSROOMS, FITNESS CENTERS, AND RECREATIONAL FACILITIES

Now that you have some ideas about distribution, let's discuss the all-important management of participants and equipment. A critical part of management is how to lift and carry a ball safely to a working space. The following is an abbreviated lesson that can be used in any setting, including fitness training or therapy, for proper lifting and carrying mechanics.

Lifting the Exercise Ball

Lesson Objective

To learn proper lifting and carrying strategies to keep people from injuring their backs.

Getting Started: Lifting and Carrying Techniques and Strategies to Get on the Ball

1. Have participants stand with feet hip-width apart and one foot slightly in front of the other. They should bend their knees and keep their backs straight while picking up an imaginary exercise ball. This is a good thing to have them practice before they get a ball.

   Emphasize bending the knees and lifting with the legs. When they are in an upright position, they can turn to change directions. Lifting and twisting simultaneously is what causes many back injuries.

2. Review these steps for safe lifting:

   • Start in the ready position.
   • Place the feet hip-width apart.
   • Put one foot slightly in front of the other.
   • Bend the knees.
   • Lift with the legs.
   • Keep the back straight.
   • Turn to face the direction you want to go when you are standing—don't twist while you are lifting!

3. Now that the participants know the proper lifting technique, they are ready to carry the ball.

   Balls should be in different areas of the room for distribution as described earlier. Reinforce and model lifting techniques.

4. Give the direction, *Start with the ball waist-high in a secured fashion while walking into open space and around the room.* Have users raise the ball over their heads and walk with it. Ask them to bring the ball back to waist level when they are tired. Emphasize the energy and effort that goes into lifting and carrying the ball without dropping it when using proper form and technique.

5. Next have participants find a self-space where they can reverse the lifting process using their legs and keeping their backs straight to place the ball on the floor. Review with participants these steps for safely lowering the ball to the floor:

- Return to the ready position.
- Place the feet hip-width apart.
- Put one foot slightly in front of the other.
- Bend the knees.
- Keep the back straight, and bend the knees more.
- Lower the ball to the ground.

6. Finally, have students place their bellies on the ball, rocking forward and backward and side to side. As students gain experience and confidence on the balls, you can expand the warm-up choices.

Lesson Extension

A favorite warm-up that engages participants is to dribble the exercise ball. The size and weight of the balls gives participants lots of feedback in terms of force needed to keep the ball waist-high and the hand position required for proper dribbling while maintaining **control**. *Control* is a cue word used by instructors to emphasize students' or clients' mastery of their movement on or with a piece of equipment. The dribbling can be practiced at different levels and directions once control has been established. Students find hand dribbling irresistible, and it also develops upper-body and core strength.

We have found that allowing people to make choices between rocking on the ball and dribbling with control is a great management tool. These are safe and fun options for getting started with the ball. Giving choices when possible and holding people accountable are key to safe, productive environments.

Important guidelines for managing the balls include the following:

1. Teach everyone a healthy respect for the balls as exercise equipment that can be dangerous if used improperly.
2. Tell your group that it is always a privilege to use exercise equipment, and most of the exercises you will be doing can be done without the ball.
3. It is so much fun to use the balls to achieve fitness goals that everyone will work hard to get and keep the privilege of using the ball.

MANAGEMENT: HOME AND OFFICE

Respectful use of the ball and careful storage will maintain good relations with coworkers and family members. Establishing guidelines that fit your personal environment are important. A YouTube video shows a person bouncing on a ball and an annoyed coworker stabbing the ball to deflate it. Lots of my friends sent this to me (Anne), and I'm glad they did. It is a topic to address because the ball could be an annoyance if used improperly. As discussed in chapter 1, our individual needs for movement to increase or maintain our productivity is something that should be talked about. Personal feelings and desires for a relaxed, calm, work environment should be respected.

The bottom line is that if you are using the exercise ball as a chair, you need to do so without disturbing others in the home, office, or school environment. If those around you are distracted, you need to discuss what the distractor factor is and modify how the ball is being used in order to maintain use without disturbing others. Small, subtle bounces and shifting your weight to gain more movement and some stretching is fine. Really big bounces and strength and stretching exercises that require larger spaces and could be a distraction to others should be saved for another time and space. Mutual respect and understanding can go a long way in preserving this fun alternative to traditional seating in a variety of settings.

Proper management of exercise balls is crucial for the successful use of the balls as a part of your program. We want to make every effort possible to help set you up to succeed. Having the right size ball for each person will help ensure success. See chapter 2, "Selection and Safety of Exercise Balls," for specifics on getting the right size ball for everyone. Easy access to a variety of different-sized balls as well as the plug puller and the dual-action hand pump mentioned in chapter 2 will have you ready to roll.

There will always be a learning curve when people get on the ball and need to balance in ways they're not used to. The benefits are huge, and the process is fun. It is a matter of putting people at ease and being sure they feel safe at whatever stage in life they may be. This means young children starting around five years old would learn in a class setting or be guided by a knowledgeable adult about safe use of the ball. Seniors should be in a safe, padded area with adequately trained professionals.

SUMMARY

Once you have the storage possibilities and ideas for ball distribution settled, you'll be on your way to managing your exercise balls with ease. In the next chapter on assessment and social and emotional challenges, you will learn more about the pair-and-share method of assessment along with other ideas to make sure you retain new things you learn. And you'll be ready to safely and confidently get on the ball with the proper mechanics. The fitness benefits will be easy to see, and the enthusiasm that comes from the natural playful nature of the ball will have you and whomever you may be working with asking for more.

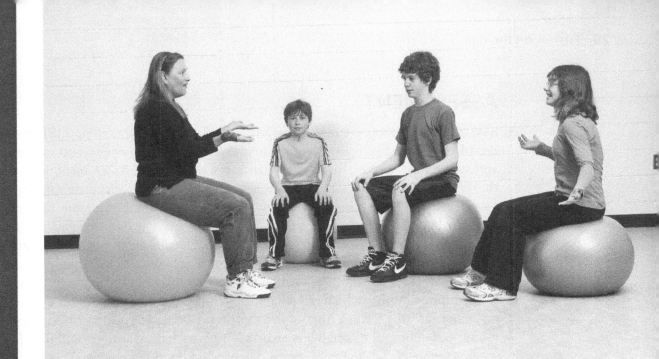

chapter four

Assessment, Proper Mechanics, and Social and Emotional Challenges

We have combined the topics of assessment, proper mechanics, and social and emotional issues in this chapter because we have found that assessment requires proper mechanics and can trigger emotional and social challenges. Assessment is a critical component of learning and working to master a skill or improve performance. Assessment provides feedback essential to the refinement of a skill. Learning proper mechanics to perform a skill ultimately allows you to be more efficient and effective. You can improve your balance, strength, and flexibility more quickly when you perform the exercise with the proper mechanics.

The final section in this chapter is about the social and emotional challenges people experience when learning new skills. Positive emotions are vital when learning and participating in physical activities and life in general. Negative emotions and social pressures have a detrimental effect on learning. Brain research on how social and emotional issues affect productivity are addressed. We encourage you to consider these factors in your working, learning, and teaching environments.

ASSESSMENT

Assessment is the act of reviewing performance. The following are four different methods of assessment: self-assessment; pair and share; partner or peer skill assessment; and supervisor, teacher, instructor, or therapist assessment. Assessment is not a test that you pass or fail. Assessment tells you what level you or those you are working with have reached in a learning progression and reviews the steps necessary to improve.

In the book *Learning Smarter: The New Science of Teaching* by Eric Jensen (2000, p. 175) the author emphasizes that self-reflection and feedback are essential to learning. Jensen discusses how important different types of specific and meaningful feedback and assessment are to skill acquisition. When new information is presented, it goes to the **hippocampus**, which is a small part of the brain that can handle only a little bit of new information at a time, or our short-term memory. The new information—if it has been delivered in small bits, makes sense, and has meaning—will then have a strong chance of sticking with you and being sent on to the **cortex**. There it can be filed away with the other things we know and can do.

Once the information is in the cortex, it can be integrated into our activities because it is now in our "hard drive," or our long-term memory (Jensen 2000). This information about our short- and long-term memory has implications to guide learning. Remember, learners can take in information only in small bits, and it must make sense and have meaning. Once all those criteria have been met, the learner needs to use the information or practice the skill before it is stored in the cortex for long-term memory.

A good example of this learning process is when you meet someone new. To remember the person's name you have to actually use it or call her by name, there has to be a context of where and why you met her, and finally she has to hold some meaning for you. I like to call this "the sticky factor," and I've broken it down to help you digest this new concept. You'll also find this in a full-page format on the CD-ROM, so if you like you can print a copy and post it where you will see it and remember to follow the guidelines when trying to learn or teach something new.

As you try out a new activity on the exercise ball, you should try to take in or give only small bits of information for each new step of how to perform the activity or exercise. Then you should assess the performance formally or informally to see if it stuck with you or your participants. Keep in mind that assessment in this situation is the ability to decide from information you have whether you are doing it right.

Specifics include the following:

- How something feels to your body—comfortable or uncomfortable.
- How the exercise looks to you. Look in a mirror and compare your posture against the photos in this book or on the bound-in CD-ROM.
- How the exercise looks to others. Demonstrate the exercise to a friend or professional to see if the movement or skill you are learning or teaching is being performed correctly.

After you perform an assessment, it's important to use the feedback you obtained:

- How did your body feel?
- How did your posture look in a mirror compared against the photos (see figure 4.1)?
- How did the exercise look to others?

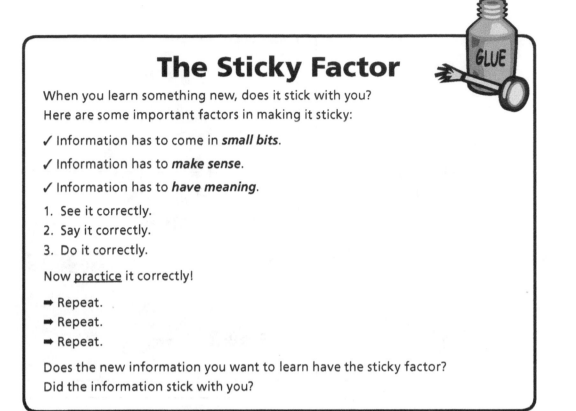

The Sticky Factor

When you learn something new, does it stick with you?
Here are some important factors in making it sticky:

✓ Information has to come in **small bits**.

✓ Information has to **make sense**.

✓ Information has to **have meaning**.

1. See it correctly.
2. Say it correctly.
3. Do it correctly.

Now <u>practice</u> it correctly!

➡ Repeat.
➡ Repeat.
➡ Repeat.

Does the new information you want to learn have the sticky factor?
Did the information stick with you?

From A. Spalding and L.E. Kelly, 2010, *Fitness on the Ball* (Champaign, IL: Human Kinetics)

Emphasis should be placed on the correct steps for completing the new activity. Then give yourself or the participants a little rest time and move on.

It is important to note that assessment can be both formal and informal. An informal assessment is an awareness and a checking in with yourself or others to be sure you are on track (see figure 4.2). The formal assessment is a written checklist of how you are performing.

Throughout this book, we provide you with a variety of informal and formal assessments, so you can choose for yourself which assessments are best for you. Once you try a few assessments we think you'll find them quick, easy, and effective. You can, of course, always design your own assessments or adapt ours. The point we want to make is that assessment is crucial to learning.

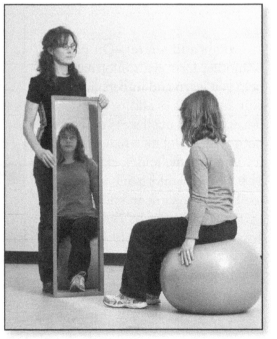

Figure 4.1 Look in a mirror and check your posture. You can do this alone, with a friend, or with a professional.

•**Self-reflection reminders**—These are things to think about in order to maintain good posture, balance, and correct mechanics. Saying or listing the critical elements in your head, out loud, or on paper will help make them stick.

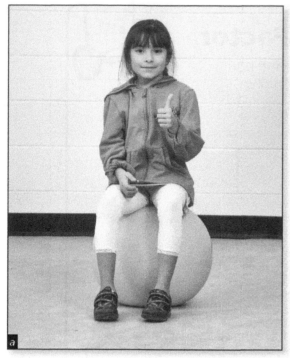

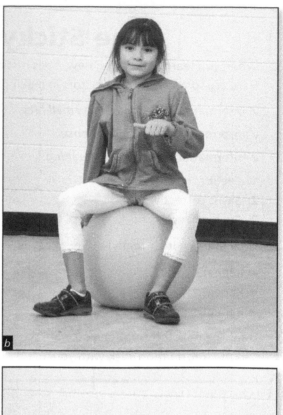

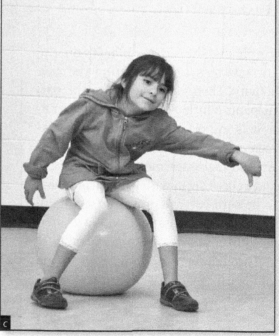

Figure 4.2 Informal assessment: *(a)* thumb up for a proper position on the ball ; *(b)* thumb sideways for a somewhat proper position on the ball; *(c)* thumb down for an incorrect position on the ball.

•**Pair and share**—On page 29 is another form with information to help you learn and understand what pair and share is and how it works. It can be used in all sorts of settings, both formal and informal. It is helpful in academic and social settings. This chunk of information is actually too big to consume in one sitting, so I usually break it up. The following are three chunks that I like to separate out: (1) how you do it, (2) active listening and paraphrasing, and (3) why you do it. Check it out and see what works best for you.

All these assessment methods will give you and your group a chance to see if the information stuck before moving on to the next exercise or activity. These assessments allow you to know how you or your group is performing. You will be able to recognize and correct errors when they occur in order to get the most out of your time on the ball.

Pair and Share

How You Do It

Turn to another person and decide who is going to share first. Groups of three also work well if you have an uneven number of people.

Active Listening and Paraphrasing

Be an **active listener** and paraphrase what you hear back to your partner or group. Active listeners

- look at you when you talk,
- nod their heads to show they are listening and engaged in what you are saying, and
- paraphrase or repeat back important bits of information that they heard.

Why You Do It

Talking about the information with other people helps remind you of what you just heard; it makes the information stick with you. Sometimes you will feel a little click and suddenly get it.

Pairing and sharing helps you remember new information and makes the information stick with you (Jensen 2000).

Remember the important factors that make the information stick with you:

✓ Information has to come in *small bits*.

✓ Information has to *make sense*.

✓ Information has to *have meaning*.

From A. Spalding and L.E. Kelly, 2010, *Fitness on the Ball* (Champaign, IL: Human Kinetics)

PROPER MECHANICS

Proper mechanics is the optimal posture or body positioning and alignment used when performing an exercise or skill. Proper mechanics allows a person to prevent injuries and achieve the desired result. In the book *Biomechanics of Musculoskeletal Injury*, Whiting and Zernicke (1998) discuss the number of people involved in accidents, including disabling injuries. They relate these injuries to **biomechanics**—the science that studies movement, posture, and body alignment and how it relates to mechanical principals.

Proper Mechanics and Newton's Laws of Motion

Remember Newton's laws of motion? You know, Sir Isaac Newton (1642-1727)! Well, here's a short review as they relate to the exercise ball.

1. A body at rest will remain at rest unless acted on by a force. (Think about an exercise ball just sitting perfectly still in the center of a room.)

2. A force acting on a body will have a reaction proportional to that exerted on the body and will respond to the force, location, and angle that it was acted on. (Think of someone coming up behind the ball and softly tapping it on the right side in order to send it to the left.)

3. For every action there is an equal and opposite reaction. (Think of the same exercise ball, and imagine the soft tap it would take to move the ball a short distance—say three feet [1 m] across the room.)

These laws are in action every time you use an exercise ball, and that is why proper mechanics and Newton's laws apply.

Think about Newton's laws and proper mechanics as you try the following mental rehearsal for getting on the ball with proper mechanics:

- Imagine slowly reaching down to stabilize an exercise ball. It is behind you—like a chair you are about to sit down on.
- You can feel the ball as you steady it using your hands.
- You slowly bend your knees while bending slightly at the waist.
- Lower yourself down slowly onto the top center of the ball.
- You are now sitting on the ball.
- Your feet are on the floor about hip-width apart.
- You engage your abdominal muscles, pulling your belly button toward your spine and elongating your torso.

There are many mechanical adjustments that happen when sitting down on a chair or a ball. The difference is that Newton's laws apply when sitting on a ball because the action involves motion. You must steady the ball before you sit on it and steady yourself while on the ball in order to sit on the ball correctly.

All these things that make you think and plan more carefully to sit on a ball safely are the same things that engage your brain in order to use the ball to exercise or use it as a chair. They are kind of like brain gymnastics. In the beginning, the basics are enough to give you a workout, and over time you add new movements to keep the brain and body humming along.

As you start to use exercise balls, you may be asking, "Is it really that important to perform the exercise correctly?" Our answer is "Absolutely!" As teachers and active people, we feel strongly that learning proper mechanics will lead to good health. We have explored a wide variety of popular exercise systems and philosophies, including Pilates, Feldenkrais, yoga, and **tai chi**. Each of these systems emphasizes proper technique and form. We integrate our knowledge of these specialized areas of study into our daily practices and this book.

Proper Mechanics and Proper Posture

Proper body mechanics refers to the way we move our bodies. Posture is an important component in body mechanics. Good **posture** generally means the spine is in a neutral or resting position. Correct body alignment is the position that provides the least stress on joints, bones, and muscles. Standing alignment consists of ear over shoulder,

shoulder over hip, hip over knee, and knee over ankle. Seated alignment is ear over shoulder, shoulder over hip, and weight on the "sitz bones," or sit bones (see figure 4.3). These positions are not static (fixed) and are individual.

Following are some tips and strategies for teaching proper mechanics:

- Perform each new skill carefully and correctly.

- Follow directions in order, and be sure the critical elements stick with you.

- Review movement vocabulary for understanding.

- Perform all skills with biomechanical correctness every time.

- Remember, posture begins in the core with the abdominal muscles contracting.

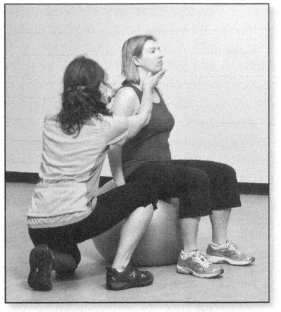

Figure 4.3 Correct body alignment seated position.

As we've explained, skill acquisition and refinement take time, practice, and feedback. Working toward learning or teaching for mastery has far-reaching implications for improved safety and performance. When you start to focus on posture and correct mechanical performance or the way you do physical things, including standing, sitting, lifting, carrying, and all physical movements, you'll feel more connected with how you move. That is the key to being conscious about your body movements and how to be an efficient and effective mover.

We've all seen injuries that were probably caused by poor form and mechanics—injuries that could have been prevented. If everyone learns the basics of good form and proper mechanics, and they begin to move more mindfully, their bodies will have enough time to learn the recently acquired skills and move them into their long-term memory or movement repertoire.

UNDERSTANDING SOCIAL AND EMOTIONAL CHALLENGES

Much of what we have read in the area of brain research emphasizes that a comfortable social and emotionally safe environment ensures optimal learning. In the book *Smart Moves: Why Learning Is Not All in Your Head*, Carla Hannaford (1995) devotes an entire chapter ("Fight or Flight: The Stress Effect on Learning") to all the different reasons that too much stress is detrimental to learning and productivity, and Daniel Goleman (1995) wrote an entire book titled *Emotional Intelligence: Why It Can Matter More Than IQ*. In his book, Goleman discusses how you can see something and your emotional response jumps in far quicker than logic. These thoughts set the stage for how each of us perceives everything from food to thunder and lightning. Depending on our past history in physical settings, we all have a very wide range of skills and abilities. Our experiences or the lack of them can make any environment where exercise occurs emotional to some degree or another. The enviroment where we try out skills should feel comfortable and nonthreatening. Anyone who has had a less than positive experience with exercise activities and balance should have a trainer, friend, therapist, or teacher with them to make the activity 100 percent safe. By that we mean physically, socially, and emotionally.

In a school environment, we establish this at the beginning of every year when we work hard to get to know every student in each of our classes. This is imperative because when we know our clients, patients, and students, we can meet their needs. As our years in the profession have shown us, each person is unique, and the key to a comfortable setting for learning is understanding their personalities and learning styles.

Here is a list of suggestions for getting to know your group:

- Take pictures of small groups, and label them with names. Now study the people and be sure you recognize them and can say hello using their names.

- Provide time for getting-to-know-you activities when the group gets to talk to each other and you. During this time, everyone shares things about themselves that feel safe to share (e.g., favorite physical activities, sports, or games that bring personal enjoyment).

- Set aside time for pair and share for everyone, including yourself. During this time, everyone talks to another person in the group about an activity they love or a fun, interesting fact about themselves.

- Be sure to greet everyone as they enter, using their names whenever possible. A warm, friendly greeting goes a long way. There is magic in knowing and remembering people's names.

- Try to give yourself time before, during, or after class to make personal contact with everyone, checking in to see how the day is going. This builds relationships that make people feel safe and comfortable (see figure 4.4).

- Provide ongoing specific feedback about performance. This can be given in many different ways including direct, specific acknowledgements; "I noticed" statements; and questions for the participant to think about. Here are some examples:

  1. *Sam, your posture looks long and strong. I can see that your ears, hips, and shoulders are all lined up.*

  2. *I noticed your alignment while sitting on the ball has improved. Are you trying to line up your ears, shoulders, and hips?*

  3. *Do you think you are increasing your core strength, and that is helping with your posture?*

- A smile goes a long way. When there is no time and all you can fit in is a smile, use it. It sends a friendly message and enhances the comfort level of any setting.

Once you know all the people in your group, it is easier to accommodate their needs. There are lots of social settings where people are shy, and as the leader or teacher it is often better to quickly assign partners and small groups instead of always asking people to find or get into partners or groups. Our recommendation

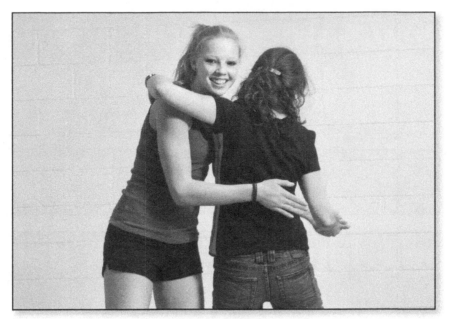

Figure 4.4 Personal contact makes a difference.

is to track your partner and small-group assignments, and be sure to carefully mix your groups for a friendly, functional, optimal learning environment. We have had students on both ends of the spectrum—shy and outgoing—thank us for these efforts, as mixing them up regularly does pay off socially. Energy put into this area is a win–win situation.

In our hometown of Boulder, Colorado, the Boulder Valley School District (BVSD) and our physical education curriculum committee understood the importance of the social and emotional needs of students. We took a stand in order to provide a safe learning environment for our students. Standard 4 in our curriculum reads as follows:

> **Standard 4: Students demonstrate safe, responsible behavior in physical education settings.** *Exhibits consideration for and cooperation with classmates and teachers (e.g., sharing turns and equipment, using supportive comments, and resolving conflicts appropriately). Works safely and productively during activity time (i.e., self-initiated or assigned task).*
>
> From the School District of Boulder, CO.

The concepts and guidelines found in the thumbnail images on page 34 are posted in our gyms. They assist us as daily reminders to teach all students socially acceptable behavior in our teaching and learning environments. These are the rules of the road in physical education classes, and when we teach them and have them posted on the walls, it helps make guidelines clear. Much in the same way that our streets and highways have speed limits, yield signs, and stop signs, these signs give all students areas of accountability and responsibility.

We invite you to use these posters, which are found on the bound-in CD-ROM, and others we mention throughout this book. Using exercise balls creates a challenging, fun, and exciting environment where individuals will be working alone, with partners, and in groups. Our goal is that everyone feels physically, socially, and emotionally safe during all learning experiences.

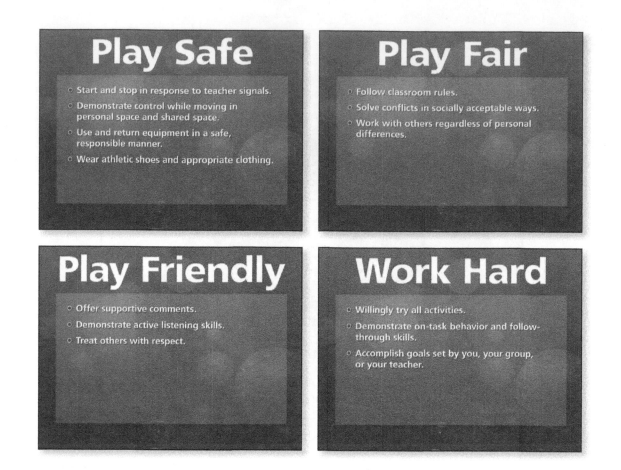

Play Safe
- Start and stop in response to teacher signals.
- Demonstrate control while moving in personal space and shared space.
- Use and return equipment in a safe, responsible manner.
- Wear athletic shoes and appropriate clothing.

Play Fair
- Follow classroom rules.
- Solve conflicts in socially acceptable ways.
- Work with others regardless of personal differences.

Play Friendly
- Offer supportive comments.
- Demonstrate active listening skills.
- Treat others with respect.

Work Hard
- Willingly try all activities.
- Demonstrate on-task behavior and follow-through skills.
- Accomplish goals set by you, your group, or your teacher.

SUMMARY

We hope this chapter has informed you about assessments, proper mechanics, and some social and emotional aspects of learning how to use an exercise ball in whatever setting you'll be in. Knowing you are doing the exercises correctly will keep you in your comfort zone. Part II is next, and you'll get all the details about basic positions, core strength exercises, and balance. Part II also includes the different components that contribute to physical fitness:

- Cardiorespiratory exercises
- Strength exercises
- Flexibility exercises

Part II is where the critical elements, clues, and cues will get you on the ball.

PART

II

Ball Exercises for Fitness: From Basic Positions to Flexibility

Part II contains activities you can do on and with the exercise ball. Chapter 5 describes the foundational positions, which you'll definitely want to review even if you have experience using exercise balls. The clues and cues are relevant and easy to remember. We think you'll like them and use them often.

Chapter 6 details the core strength that is required for good posture. It presents guidance on building muscular strength and endurance in your core so that you can easily perform daily tasks and recreational activities. Chapter 7 covers balance, and you'll find activities that are both fun and challenging to get you on the ball and beyond. Cardiorespiratory fitness exercises are covered in chapter 8. Imagine getting your heart pumping a little faster from your chair, ball, or active seating device. Exercises for muscular strength are covered in chapter 9, so you're sure to increase whole-body strength using this one piece of equipment. Flexibility exercises are presented in chapter 10. These exercises will help you improve your range of motion and maintain that reach that you need in order to become and stay active. Think *functional fitness*—the ability to perform your daily activities and chores without stress and strain.

Chapters 5 through 10 bring you explanations, critical elements, clues, and cues so you can integrate specific exercises into your everyday life, whether you're a beginner or an advanced athlete. You'll soon see and feel the improvements in your fitness level.

five

Basic Positions

• •

In this chapter, we explain the basic positions for working on an exercise ball. If you or your group has not used a ball previously, this is the place to start. Other readers can review this material to reacquaint themselves with the basic positions for working on an exercise ball. Most of the explanations for exercises in the remaining chapters in this part of the book will start with one of these positions. No extensive explanation of the starting positions will be repeated in the other chapters.

The idea of basic body positions comes out of an effort to provide a common basic vocabulary for all users and to have a safe environment and time on task in the physical education setting. *Time on task* is a phrase frequently used in the teaching profession to emphasize the need to have students actively engaged and not waiting. While the instructor is getting each person on an appropriate ball, the other students will experiment (often unknowingly and unsafely) unless they have been given a safe task to begin trying. Demonstrating comfortable, safe exercises starting on the belly gives everyone time to explore safely while the instructor focuses on safe distribution and sizing of the balls.

We include an assessment for your use along with each exercise. These assessments appear on the bound-in CD-ROM at the back of this book in the Assessment Forms folder and include a number that corresponds with the number found at the beginning of each exercise in this book. These assessments can be used for self-assessment, teacher observation, and peer assessment. Using these assessments helps

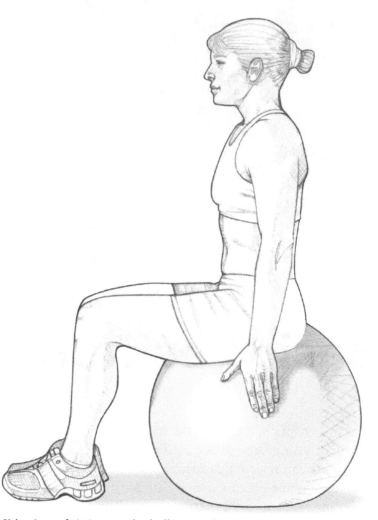

Side view of sitting on the ball correctly.

all users (individuals, students, and clients) to understand the importance of proper alignment and performing the positions correctly. By reflecting on their own ability and helping a partner reflect on their ability, students become teachers and improve their own skill and understanding. All exercise ball users are

- learners,
- coaches, and
- teachers.

We have placed the basic positions for doing an exercise in a progression that is safe and low to the floor. A **progression** is a principle of training. To improve a fitness component, exercise must gradually get more difficult. The progression in this chapter is for primary students (K-2), novice users, challenged students, people with disabilities, and those who need experience with the ball because the instructor has assessed that their self-control and risk aversion behaviors are not well developed.

Prone Position (Belly on the Ball)

Vocabulary

- elongated
- mindful
- prone
- weight transfer

Instructions

Have everyone complete the following movements:

1. Place the ball on the floor, and kneel on the floor behind it, keeping hands on the ball (see figure 5.1*a*).

2. Lean forward, placing belly and chest on the ball in a **prone** position. Keep feet and knees on the floor at first (see figure 5.1*b*).

3. Rock forward and backward, pushing and pulling gently with feet and knees. See how **elongated** you can make your spine while keeping feet and knees on the floor. Individuals who achieve the correct position should demonstrate for others (see figure 5.1*c*).

4. Next, push knees off the floor and reach forward with hands, placing them on the floor. This position looks like a spider with support (see figure 5.1*d*).

5. Rock slowly forward and back, and feel the **weight transfer** between the feet and hands (see figure 5.1, *e* and *f*). *Note:* This is a safe, comfortable way to begin. Use the word **mindful** to help people slow down and allow their brains and bodies to work in a coordinated fashion. Being on the ball is a coordinated movement that will have a different difficulty factor for each person. The person who thinks other activities are easy may be the same one who ends up on his head if he is not coached to move slowly and mindfully.

6. Next try side-to-side rocking (left hand and left foot to right hand and right foot). Stress the weight transfer of the movement (see figure 5.1, *g* and *h*).

7. Ask who can combine the two weight transfer movements: forward and backward, side to side, or varying combinations of hand and foot lifts to test their balance.

Assessment

The assessment form for this exercise appears as a full-size form for easy printing on the bound-in CD-ROM at the back of this book.

(continued)

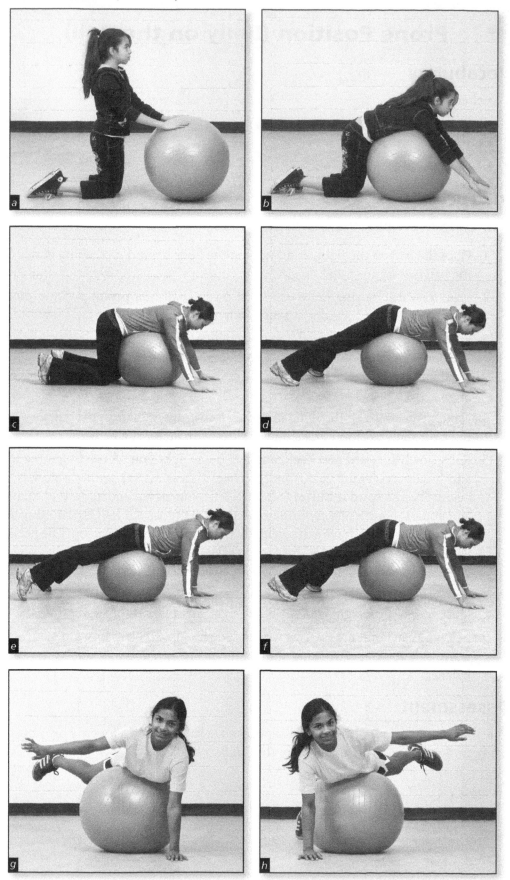

Figure 5.1 *(a)* Kneeling behind the ball; *(b)* placing chest and belly on the ball; *(c)* rocking forward and back with knees on floor; *(d)* spider; *(e and f)* transferring weight forward and back; *(g and h)* transferring weight side to side.

Seated on the Ball (Bottom on the Ball)

Next we sit on the ball. We purposely did not start seated because we want people to focus on the importance of posture, or sitting on the ball correctly, when participating in a variety of fun exercises. Having used the ball in the prone position gets everyone off to a safe start.

Instructions

Have everyone complete the following movements:

1. Stand in front of the exercise ball, closely enough for calves to touch the ball. Keep ball in place with one hand.

2. Lower your body slowly and with control into a seated position. Tell everyone, *Remember not to plop because the ball rebounds like a trampoline.*

3. Feet should be approximately shoulder-width apart and parallel (see figure 5.2, *a* and *b*).

4. *Keep feet on the floor.* At this point, a number of people will be struggling with balance. Explain that a wider stance is more stable (demonstrate by moving your feet wider apart) and that a narrower stance is less stable (slide your feet together and wobble a bit). *Shoulder width is the starting position for feet, and if you need more stability, then it is okay to move feet a bit wider.* Emphasize that we are challenging our balance when working on the ball and that each person will gradually move their feet closer as they are ready.

Note: There will always be those people who are capable of sitting on the ball and behaving and those people who are clowning about and being wild. We emphasize the necessity of following directions exactly. If anyone is not following directions,

(continued)

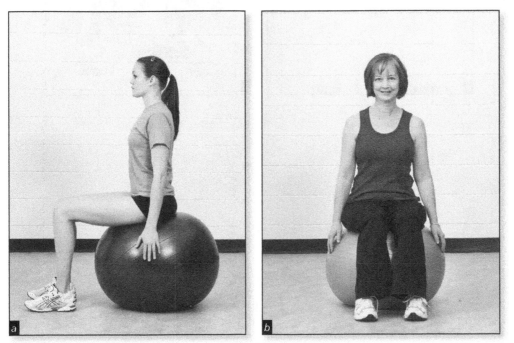

Figure 5.2 *(a)* Seated properly on the ball; *(b)* feet position.

Seated on the Ball   *(continued)*

that person loses the opportunity to use the ball. Tell your group, *Every person learns differently. Some like to work with the equipment, and others benefit from watching. Which type of learner are you?*

Assessment

Since writing the first edition of this book, *Kids on the Ball*, we have found new ways of teaching this skill. We tell students, *Place two fists between the knees or a hand width (thumb to pinkie) between the feet to check the leg position* (see figure 5.3, *a* and *b*). Non-verbal cues are very valuable when getting a large group to sit on the ball quickly and quietly and with proper form. This also helps with the concept of training the brain to focus. A poster or an overhead with an illustration of sitting on the ball correctly is critical for your visual learners, and either of these can be created using the illustration from page 38 and from the bound-in CD-ROM.

The assessment form for this exercise appears as a full-size form for easy printing on the bound-in CD-ROM at the back of this book.

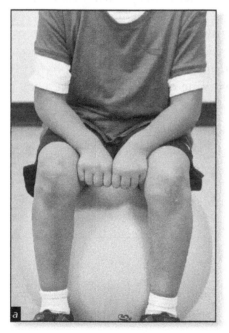

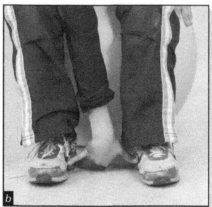

Figure 5.3   *(a)* Measuring stance with fists; *(b)* measuring stance with thumb and pinkie finger.

Side on the Ball

Instructions

Have everyone complete the following movements:

1. Kneel on the floor with the ball at the side, hand on the ball (see figure 5.4a).
2. Lean hip and lay side of torso on the ball, sliding the hand and arm over the ball (see figure 5.4b).
3. Straighten top leg until it extends straight from hip (see figure 5.4c).
4. Raise top arm to ceiling. Balance for 5 to 10 seconds (see figure 5.4d).
5. Repeat on other side.

Note: This position takes major focus, strength, and balance and challenges most people. It should be done slowly, and an attempt should be made to hold the position for three or more counts. Repeating this balance exercise is very important, and most people will find one side more challenging than the other.

This is a good time to talk about core strength and dominant sides of the body. Ask the people in your group if they are right or left handed, and remind them regularly that when they notice one side of the body is weaker or movements are more difficult or wobbly, it is a sign they need to work that side harder to help it catch up and balance out both sides of the body.

(continued)

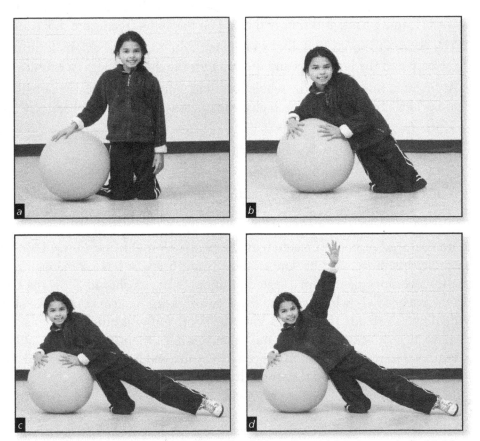

Figure 5.4 *(a)* Kneeling with ball at side; *(b)* kneeling with torso on ball; *(c)* side on ball with leg extended; *(d)* side on ball with leg extended and arm to ceiling.

Side on the Ball *(continued)*

Current trends in fitness focus on core strength. Our core is where all our movements originate, and when the core is strong we feel more stable. Once people understand this concept, and you've discussed it in relation to posture, everyday activities, and achievement in movement and sport, they will be conscious and aware of it in themselves and others.

Assessment

The assessment form for this exercise appears as a full-size form for easy printing on the bound-in CD-ROM at the back of this book.

 # Tabletop (Back on the Ball)

Vocabulary

• scapulae

Instructions

Have everyone complete the following movements:

1. From the seated position with hands lightly on the ball, walk feet forward while leaning back and rolling the ball on the spine (see figure 5.5, *a* and *b*).

2. The position should look like a table, with the torso and thighs forming the tabletop and the lower legs and the ball forming the table legs (see figure 5.5*c*).

3. At first it is fine to have the whole back and spine supported by the ball. This looks like a backbend and will give a marvelous stretch to the back (see figure 5.5*d*).

4. Assess to see if the students can keep
   • feet shoulder-width apart (or closer),
   • **scapulae** (shoulder blades) on the ball, and
   • hips lifted so there is a straight line from knees to shoulders.

Use an overhead or poster created with the photos from the bound-in CD-ROM to demonstrate this move, and be sure to show your group, or have someone demonstrate, the slow movement from a seated position. Students should allow the ball to roll up the back slowly while walking feet forward, keeping arms out to the side or reaching down to steady themselves from the floor. You will quickly see that some people have incredible core strength and balance, while others will struggle and need to be reminded to go slowly and may need to stay in a modified position until a later time when they have built up the strength and balance.

Assessment

The assessment form for this exercise appears as a full-size form for easy printing on the bound-in CD-ROM at the back of this book.

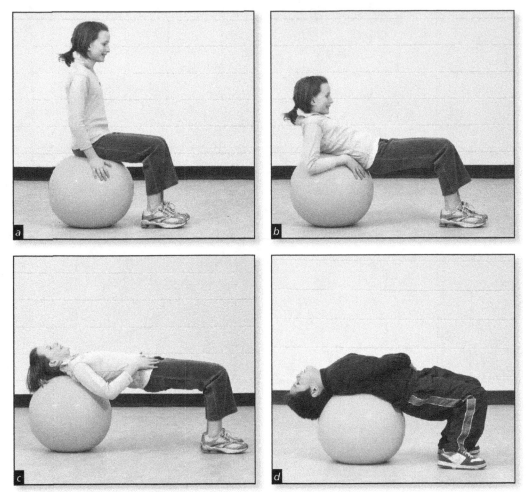

Figure 5.5 *(a)* Beginning tabletop: hands on ball; *(b)* beginning tabletop: rolling ball down spine; *(c)* correct tabletop position; *(d)* arched tabletop.

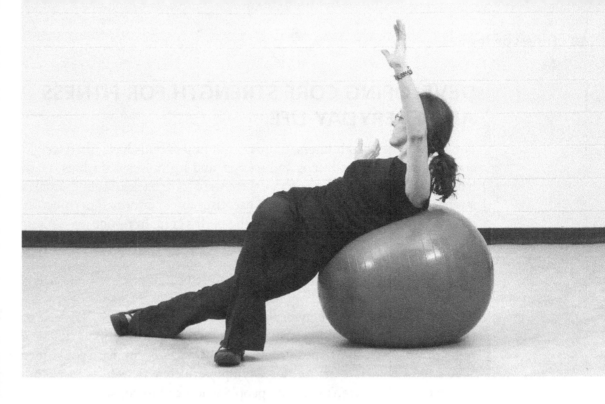

Core Strength Exercises

· ·

The core consists of all the muscles in the torso, from the small deep muscles in the pelvis, back, chest, and abdominal area to the more well-known larger ones, including the abdominals, trapezius, pectoralis major, and latissimus dorsi. Core strength is the basis for all movement and is literally the center, or core, of our daily lives. A weak core can result in back and other injuries, while a strong core helps people maintain balance and better perform strength and flexibility activities (which include daily activities, physical activity, and sport activities).

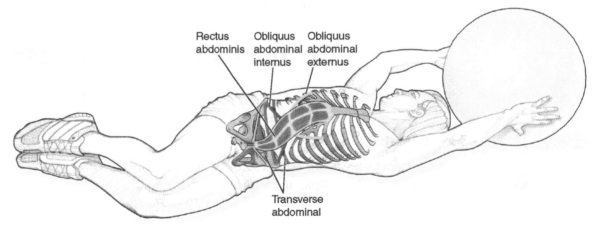

Rectus abdominis

Obliquus abdominal internus

Obliquus abdominal externus

Transverse abdominal

Muscles used during core strength exercises.

DEVELOPING CORE STRENGTH FOR FITNESS AND EVERYDAY LIFE

For a long time, weightlifters, trainers, and fitness buffs have lifted weights to make arm muscles, such as biceps and triceps, and leg muscles, such as quadriceps and hamstrings, stronger. For the torso, there were some back and abdominal exercises to strengthen these muscles, but those exercises were performed perfunctorily without much insight into the importance of the body's core. In recent years, there has been an increasing emphasis on developing the strength of the torso, or core, because it truly is the origin of our movement.

Athletes especially need core training to reduce injuries. When the core is weak, the athlete uses other parts of the body, specifically the legs and arms, to produce power and speed. This often results in joint and muscle injuries because the muscles shorten from the constant repetitions, and the range of motion (ROM) of joints is reduced. In effect, sport-specific muscle imbalances occur, with consequent injuries.

A strong core is essential for Olympic athletes as well as weekend warriors. However, athletes aren't the only people who need to consider their core strength. In fact, everybody needs a strong core, from toddlers to seniors. Through exercises with exercise balls, toddlers can improve their motor skills earlier and become more balanced walkers. Seniors can improve their balance and prevent life-threatening falls through core strength training. Core strength training improves the efficient functioning of everyone's musculoskeletal system and maintains the ideal posture that is essential for movement.

EFFECTIVELY TRAINING YOUR CORE

To effectively train the core, you need a variety of exercises that target the muscles of the torso from many different angles and planes of motion. In addition, the exercises should closely approximate and target functional, everyday movements and be dynamic rather than static.

The exercise ball helps you achieve the necessary functional, dynamic exercise you need in order to strengthen your core. The round, mobile, and unstable surface of the exercise ball forces the core muscles to work harder to maintain balance. The exercise ball requires you to work more muscles at the same time, and the exercises are therefore better and more efficient at improving functioning.

Basic Core Strength Exercises

The following exercises are for everyone who wants a stronger core. They form the basic exercises that are the beginning of core strength for the back and abdominal muscles.

Assessment

The assessment forms for these exercises appear as full-size forms for easy printing on the bound-in CD-ROM at the back of this book.

Vocabulary

• supine

Instructions

Have everyone complete the following movements:

1. Starting position: Lie on back (**supine**) on the floor with the ball under the calves of both legs, which will put the thighs perpendicular to the floor (see figure 6.1*a*).

2. Keeping abdominal muscles contracted, lift arms straight above shoulders. Make scissor motions, alternating arms back and forth for 20 repetitions, touching thighs lightly (head remains on floor; see figure 6.1*b*).

3. Repeat 20 times, alternately lifting one leg slightly off ball and touching with one hand as the arms scissor (see figure 6.1*c*).

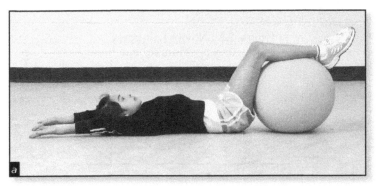

Figure 6.1 Dead Bug: *(a)* starting position; *(b)* arm scissor; *(c)* touching arms to lifted leg.

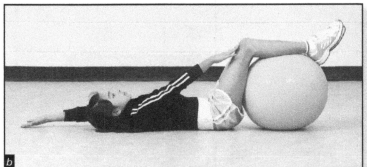

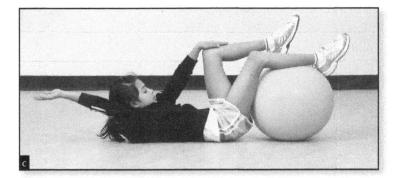

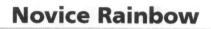

Instructions

Have everyone complete the following movements:

1. Starting position: Lie on back on the floor with the ball under the calves of both legs, which will put the thighs perpendicular to the floor.
2. Contract abdominal muscles as you use your legs to roll the ball to the side (see figure 6.2).
3. When you feel your obliques engage, you have rolled the ball far enough. Bring back to original position (center).
4. Repeat on other side.

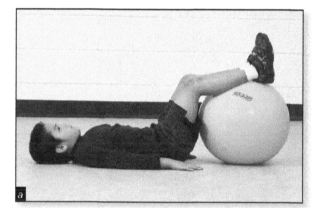

Figure 6.2 Novice Rainbow: *(a)* starting position; *(b)* ball rolled off center.

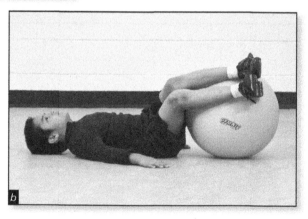

Instructions

Have everyone complete the following movements:

1. Starting position: Lie prone on the ball, weight on feet and hands off floor (see figure 6.3*a*).

2. Contract back muscles, lift arms to ear level, and raise back to form a straight line with feet and shoulders (see figure 6.3*b*).

3. Hold for two counts, and return slowly to start (controlled, not a collapse).

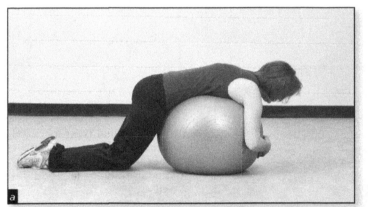

Figure 6.3 Back Extensions: *(a)* starting position; *(b)* ending position.

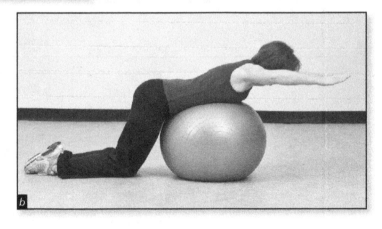

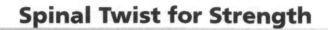

Spinal Twist for Strength

Instructions

Have everyone complete the following movements:

1. Starting position: Lie supine on floor with knees bent and thighs perpendicular to floor. Hold ball on floor with hands and arms extended (see figure 6.4*a*).

2. Slowly move both legs to one side without touching the floor. At the same time, roll the ball in the opposite direction and turn head to look at the ball (see figure 6.4*b*).

3. Bring knees back to original position.

4. Repeat on opposite side.

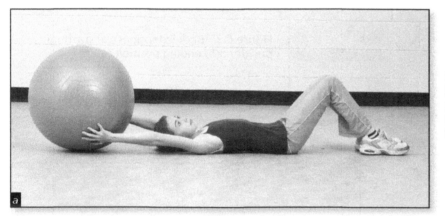

Figure 6.4 Spinal Twist for Strength: *(a)* starting position; *(b)* knees toward floor and use abdominals to guide legs and the ball.

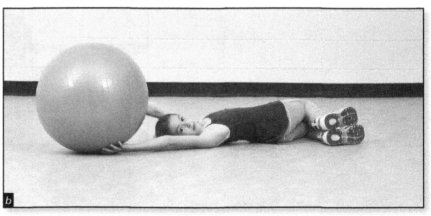

Active Sitting Exercises

Active sitting is generally considered using the exercise ball as a chair or using an inflated disc as an active seating device. The benefits are covered in chapter 1. Two of the biggest benefits are better posture and core strength. It is difficult to slump and sit comfortably on the ball. Seated posture becomes more erect because the spine is stacked like blocks, and the spinal muscles become engaged along with the abdominal muscles. However, sitting on the ball can be tiring at first and should be alternated with chair sitting, gradually spending more time on the ball and less in a chair. Following are some exercises to accompany active sitting or desk exercises.

Assessment

The assessment forms for these exercises appear as full-size forms for easy printing on the bound-in CD-ROM at the back of this book.

Forward and Back

Instructions

Have everyone complete the following movements:

1. Starting position: Sit correctly on the ball (see figure 5.2a on page 41).
2. With hips, roll ball forward toward feet (do not move feet) (see figure 6.5a).
3. Next use hips to roll the ball backward (see figure 6.5b).
4. Repeat slowly and gently 5 to 10 times, gently loosening pelvic area and spine.

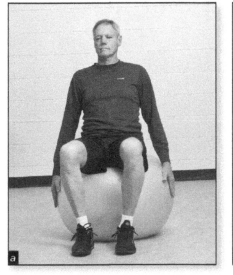
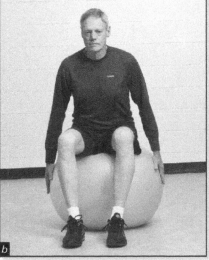

Figure 6.5 Forward and Back: *(a)* rolling ball forward toward feet; *(b)* rolling ball backward.

Instructions

Have everyone complete the following movements:

1. Starting position: Sit correctly on the ball (see figure 5.2*a* on page 41).
2. Rock ball side to side by rolling the ball with the hips (see figure 6.6).

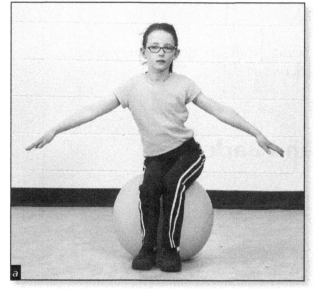 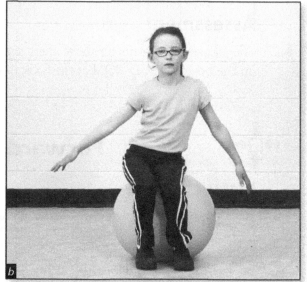

Figure 6.6 Side to Side.

Hula

Instructions

Have everyone complete the following movements:

1. Starting position: Sit correctly on the ball (see figure 5.2*a* on page 41).
2. Combine Forward and Back with Side to Side and rotate the ball in a circle: forward, side, back, side, and forward (see figure 6.7).
3. After three to five circles, go in the other direction.

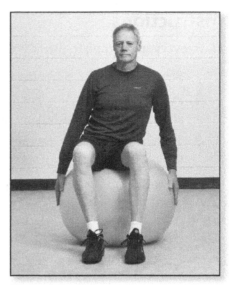

Figure 6.7 Hula.

Shoulder Shrug

Instructions

Have everyone complete the following movements:

1. Starting position: Sit correctly on the ball (see figure 5.2*a* on page 41).
2. Hang arms down by sides and away from the ball. Rotate arms and shoulders forward, then backward. Relax scapulae on the forward rotation, and squeeze scapulae on backward rotation.
3. Next lift shoulders toward ears, and then drop shoulders (see figure 6.8). Repeat five times.
4. Circle shoulders backward five times, and then circle forward five times.

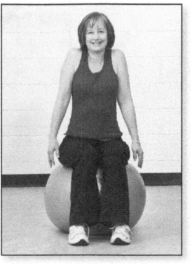

Figure 6.8 Shoulder Shrug.

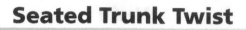

Instructions

Have everyone complete the following movements:

1. Starting position: Sit correctly on the ball (see figure 5.2*a* on page 41).
2. Place right forearm in front of waist, with hand by left side. Place left forearm at back of waist, with hand at right side.
3. Turn head to the left, looking over left shoulder and twisting spine gently. Hold for a few seconds, then return to start (see figure 6.9).
4. Reverse arm positions and twist to right.

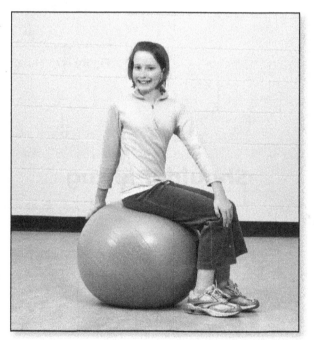

Figure 6.9 Seated Trunk Twist.

OTHER CORE EXERCISES

All exercises on the ball involve the core because of the need to stabilize the ball. The exercises earlier in this chapter are just the beginning of the journey. Because we have organized the following chapters by categories (balance, strength, and flexibility), we will refer you to those chapters now. Everyone will have a different experience with the different exercise categories as well as within each category. Your strength or weakness will depend on your regular daily activities, your level of participation in different sports, and your fitness level. Anyone and everyone can gain from exercises on the ball. Try out the first exercises in each category to find out your status. Then progress to the exercises that are more difficult. All exercises in each category have been ordered in a progression from easy to more difficult.

APPLYING CORE STRENGTH TRAINING TO SPECIFIC SPORTS

For every sport there is a training program that can maximize performance. The exercises in this book will meet the general requirements of all sports: balance, strength, and flexibility. As you learn the exercises and become familiar with the purpose of each exercise, you will learn how your body responds. Being mindful of how your body reacts will be your best guide to developing your own unique program. What exercise is hardest for you? Repeat that exercise for a second or third set. That will strengthen those muscles required for that exercise. Gradually, you will find that exercise is easier. Is there a particular side of your body that is weak or weaker than the other side? Start your sets on that particular side, and then return to that side for a little extra work on those specific muscles.

As you begin to learn more about your specific muscles through core strength training, analyze your performance during your sport to determine where your muscle imbalances occur. Choose strength and flexibility exercises from this book that will help you offset these imbalances. For example, if you are a runner, your legs get a tremendous workout. To prevent muscle shortening you will need to religiously stretch the hip, knee, and ankle joints to maintain your ROM. In addition, core training in the tabletop position introduced in chapter 5 will be invaluable for improving your balance and strength.

The following are brief discussions of various sport applications of core training, balance, strength, and flexibility exercises on the exercise ball.

- **Golf:** You think you need a new set of clubs to improve your drives, but actually, you just need to strengthen your core to improve your balance and flexibility. And it will cost less than new clubs. Focus on core strength (abdominal and back) exercises.

- **Soccer:** Core strength will improve balance and agility necessary to maneuver around other players and control the ball while appearing to be off balance. Stretches for **hip flexors** and **piriformis** muscles will improve play. Also focus on hamstring and quadriceps exercises for legs and abdominal and back strength exercises.

- **Basketball:** Core training will strengthen the torso for aerial moves, including blocking shots and making jump shots, and improve shooting accuracy because the core will be so stable. As in soccer, a stronger core will also improve agility—or the ability to quickly change direction—necessary for deceptive fakes. Focus on abdominal and back strength exercises. Do both hamstring exercises and quadriceps strength exercises for the legs.

- **Volleyball:** Hitting in volleyball takes place off the ground and requires a strong core for maintaining balance and powering a forceful hit. A wild, unbalanced attack will not have the power necessary to score a kill. Focus on abdominal strength exercises for hitting, along with spinal twisting strength. Do standing lunges for quadriceps strength for jumping and landing.
- **Football:** NFL teams to peewee football need strong, balanced players. Every position benefits from core training, and many NFL teams use exercise balls as a part of their training regimens.

Advanced Core Strength Exercises

The exercises in this section are examples of more difficult core strength exercises like those you will encounter in the later chapters. These exercises can be attempted by people who have experience with the dynamic nature of the exercise ball. These would be considered intermediate-level exercises and should be attempted slowly during the learning phase.

Assessment

The assessment forms for these exercises appear as full-size forms for easy printing on the bound-in CD-ROM at the back of this book.

Torso Turners

Instructions

Have everyone complete the following movements:

1. Starting position: Place your belly on the ball, with weight on the feet and arms off the floor (see figure 6.10*a*).
2. Place one hand on the floor, raise other arm toward the ceiling, and roll slowly onto your side (see figure 6.10*b*).
3. Continue to roll in the same direction until your back is on the ball (like table-top) (see figure 6.10*c*) and then your other side (see figure 6.10*d*) and finally your belly (see figure 6.10*e*).
4. Now repeat, going in the other direction. This is a wonderful exercise for balance, coordination, and whole-brain engagement.

Variation

Do Torso Turners without using the hands on the floor.

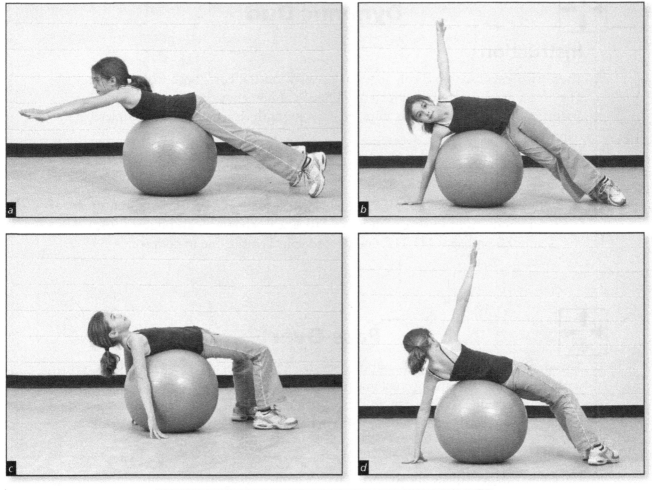

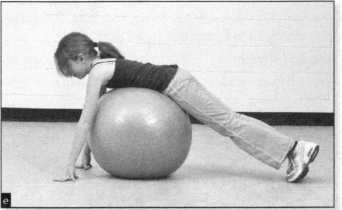

Figure 6.10 Torso Turners: *(a)* starting position; *(b)* phase two; *(c)* tabletop phase on back; *(d)* tabletop phase on side; *(e)* tabletop phase on belly.

Dynamic Duo

Instructions

These two exercises go nicely together to work on the core, both front and back. They are a great combination for a quick break at home, work, or school to increase attention and focus as well as improve core strength. Have everyone complete the following movements:

1. Seated Mini Curl-Up: See exercise description and figure 9.15 on page 123 in chapter 9.
2. Push-ups: See exercise descriptions of Rocking Push-Up, Belly Button Push-Up, and Thigh Push-Up on pages 110-112 in chapter 9 and figures 9.1, 9.2, and 9.3 on pages 111-112, and choose your favorite one to perform.

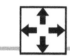

Pass Over

This duo can have a variety of combinations, from Pass Over and Pass Over–Roll Over with the hip lift, hamstring combination, and hummers. We like offering people lots of exercise options so they can do these alone or with a friend. The beginning and advanced choices also help to keep everyone in their comfort zone.

Instructions

Have everyone complete the following movements:

1. Starting position: Lie on your back with knees bent, feet on the floor, and the exercise ball overhead in hands (see figure 6.11a).
2. Lift the ball, and straighten the legs toward the ceiling (see figure 6.11b).
3. Transfer the ball from hands to feet, and lower the ball to the ground (see figure 6.11c).
4. Reverse the order, and pass the ball back to the hands. Repeat.

Variations

- **Individual Pass Over–Roll Over:** Share these instructions with your group: Same as the original Pass Over exercise, except when the ball is in your hands, roll over to touch it to the right and then the left side of your body (see figure 6.12a). When the ball is held with your feet, you will again roll over to touch the ball to the right and then the left side (see figures 6.12b-d). Repeat.
- After you have completed Individual Pass Over–Roll Over, try it with a friend. These extensions are a fun social mixer, and some people may choose to continue alone while others will go on to find a friend and then a group of three. It's all about choices in terms of meeting everyone's needs.

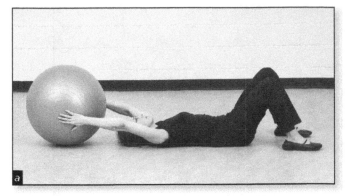

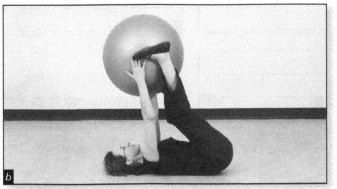

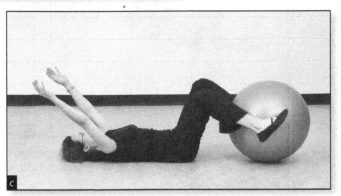

Figure 6.11 Pass Over: *(a)* starting position; *(b)* passing the ball to the feet; *(c)* lowering the ball to the floor.

- **Partner Pass Over–Roll Over:** Share these instructions with your group: Lie beside a friend. One of you has the ball in your hands. Roll first to the side that is open, and touch the ball to the floor; when you come back up you will pass the ball to you partner's hands. Your partner will roll over and touch the ball to her open side and then come back up and pass it back to you. You will then pass it to your feet and repeat the exercise using the feet (see figure 6.13, *a-e*).

- **Group of Three Pass Over–Roll Over:** Share these instructions with your group: Lie side by side with two friends, and do the Partner Pass Over–Roll Over exercise, except when you are in the middle you will always be passing to someone instead of touching the ball to the ground. You can rotate who is in the middle so everyone gets a turn (see figure 6.14).

(continued)

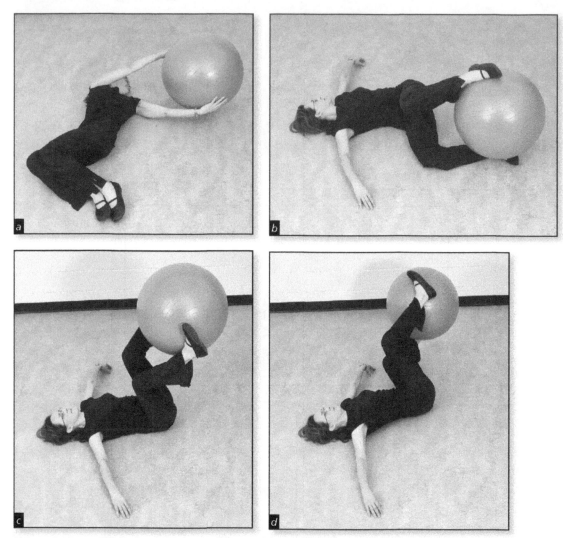

Figure 6.12 Individual Pass Over–Roll Over: *(a)* with ball in hands, touching ball to right and left sides of body; *(b-d)* with ball held by feet, touching ball to the right and left side.

After trying some of these exercises, you can finish with the following to complete the Dynamic Duos:

- Hip Lift (see figure 9.37 on page 144 in chapter 9)
- Hamstring Combination (see figure 9.38 on page 145 in chapter 9)
- Hummers (perform Hamstring Combination without lowering hips)

As you become more comfortable and familiar with ball exercises, you and your students or clients will probably come up with many more fun combinations to improve core strength.

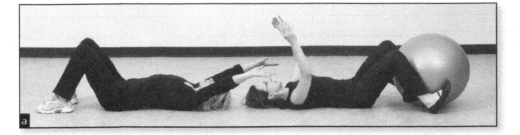

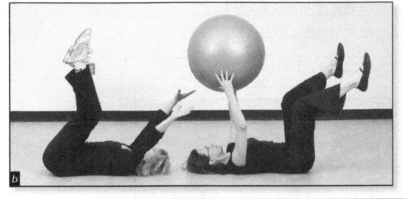

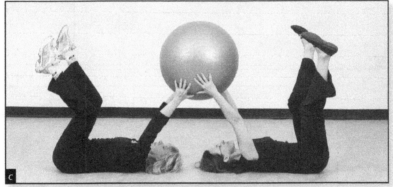

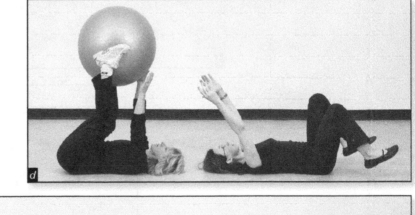

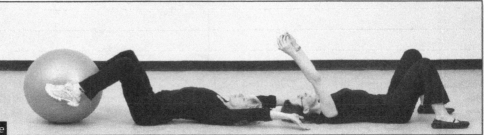

Figure 6.13 Partner Pass Over–Roll Over: *(a)* one partner begins with exercise ball between feet; *(b)* first person passes ball to own hands; *(c)* first person transfers ball to partner's hands; *(d)* second person passes the ball to own feet; *(e)* second person touches ball to floor.

(continued)

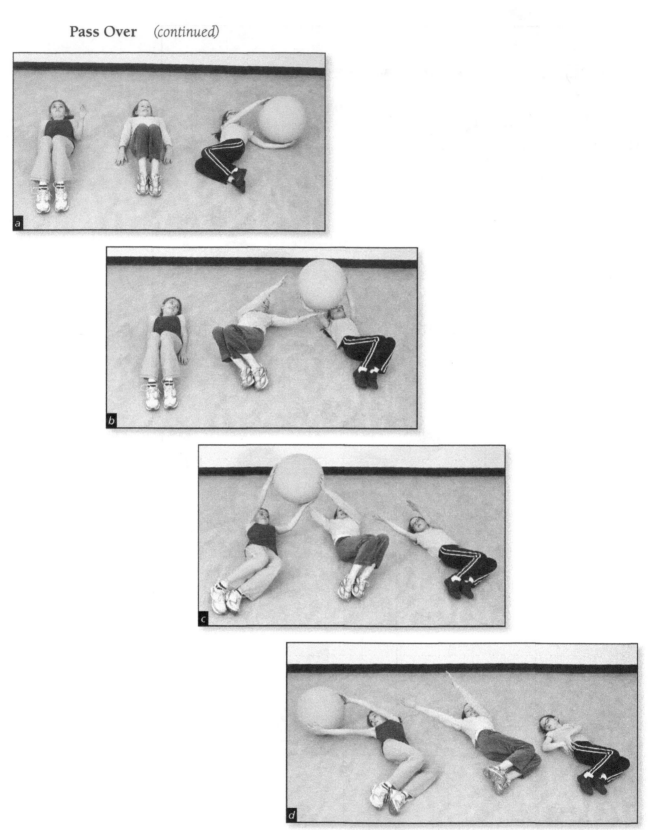

Figure 6.14 Group of Three Pass Over–Roll Over: *(a)* first person starts with ball held in hands and touches floor; *(b)* first person passes the ball to the second person who drops knees in opposite direction; *(c)* as the second person passes the ball to the third person, the second person drops her knees to the other side; *(d)* the third person touches the ball to the floor and drops her knees to the opposite side.

Balance Exercises

· ·

Balance is a skill that is often neglected because we take it for granted. That is a mistake because balance is critical for everyday activities in addition to physical activity. It is not just a skill that gymnasts or high-wire walkers need. Every day we encounter situations where we are a little off balance and instantly recover. Improving this skill, by practicing balance and honing the skill, will protect us from falls or allow us to fall more safely, as well as serve as the basis for improving performance in sports. Balance is a key component of athleticism, and everyone can develop a higher level of balance.

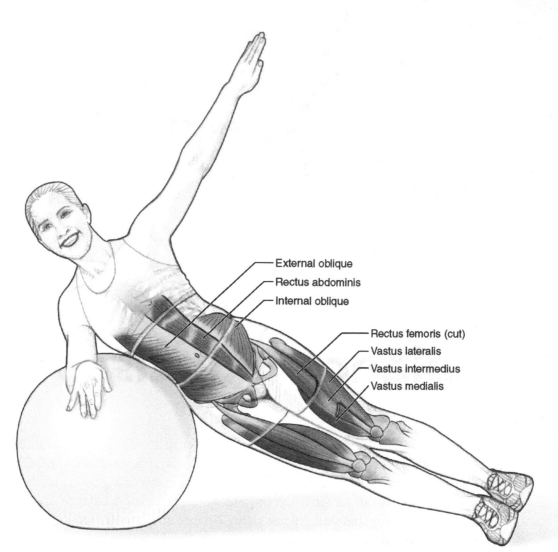

Muscles used during balance exercises.

Balance Vocabulary Exercise

Vocabulary

- base of support
- center of gravity
- dynamic balance
- gravity
- off balance
- on balance
- static balance
- steady
- wobbly

Instructions

1. Put the vocabulary terms on strips of paper with die-cut letters or 72-point font on the computer.

2. When introducing a new vocabulary word, follow these steps.
   - Use it in a sentence: *Today we are going to work on balance.*
   - Emphasize its importance by saying the word alone: *balance.*
   - Ask the class to repeat the word out loud: *balance.*
   - Show them the written word. Tell students, *See, this is how it is spelled. Spell it out loud with me: b-a-l-a-n-c-e.*
   - Ask the students to define the term, or provide the definition for them.

3. Students will have heard the word, said the word, and seen the word. Now, as they do the exercise—in this instance, practice balance—their brains have four ways that help it remember the concept (this is the sticky factor that we discussed earlier in this book).

4. At the end of class, review the vocabulary words. Tell the students, *We learned about* **base of support, center of gravity, dynamic balance, static balance, gravity, on balance,** *and* **off balance** [and any other words you reviewed]. *Raise your hand if you can tell me one of the concepts we practiced.*

5. Dismiss students to line up by who can tell you one of the vocabulary words.

Balance Activity to Accompany Balance Vocabulary

Share the following activity with your group:

1. What am I standing on? (two feet)

2. Yes, that is my base of support.

3. Now change the size of your base of support; make it larger. Can you stay on balance if it gets too wide? When you start to fall, then you are off balance. Balance with the widest base of support you can, and be on balance. Are you **steady** (not moving)? Or are you **wobbly** (shaky and wiggly)?

4. Repeat the exercise, changing to a small base of support. When students are comfortable with the balance vocabulary words, they are ready to move on to the balance activities with the exercise ball.

Exercise Benefits

This exercise reinforces experiential understanding of balance vocabulary.

Variations

Add the concept of shape to a follow-up lesson.

Hints for Various Age Levels

Appropriate for all levels.

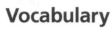

One-Leg Balance

Vocabulary

The vocabulary is the same for all the balance exercises and should be reinforced in each lesson.

Instructions

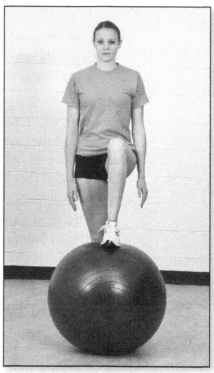

1. Starting position: Stand behind the ball so that the ball is in front of the right leg.
2. Support the body weight on the left leg while placing the right foot lightly on top of the ball (see figure 7.1).
3. Write the letters of the alphabet with the foot touching the ball. *Note:* There is no weight placed on the ball by the right foot.

Exercise Benefits

This exercise challenges and strengthens the muscles in the foot and ankle.

The small muscles of the foot and ankle must respond to the slight imbalance caused by moving the ball while standing on one leg. The **proprioceptors** in these muscles get a workout as they give feedback to the body, helping maintain balance.

Figure 7.1 One-Leg Balance: alphabet writing.

Variations

Be sure all weight is transferred to the supporting leg, then lift the writing leg, and pull in abdominal muscles and stand tall. See how long you can balance on one foot with the other leg held above the ball.

Hints for Various Age Levels

- **K-2:** Use alphabet letters on cards to help with tracing the letters. Do two or three letters with one leg, and then switch to the other leg. Gradually increase the amount of time spent on one leg.

- **3-5:** Do one-third to one-half of the alphabet at a time. Have the class say each letter out loud as they begin to write it.

- **6-12:** Write the whole alphabet before switching legs. (Even adults have difficulty with this.) Use large movements to challenge balance. Remind students to immediately remove the foot from the ball if they begin to lose their balance. Recognizing when they start to go off balance is as important as trying to stay on balance.

Assessment

The assessment form for this exercise appears as a full-size form for easy printing on the bound-in CD-ROM at the back of this book.

Seated Balances

Vocabulary

The vocabulary is the same for all the balance exercises and should be reinforced in each lesson.

Exercise Benefits

Benefits of these seated balance exercises include engaging and strengthening the following muscles:

- Quadriceps (rectus femoris, vastus lateralis, vastus medialis, and vastus intermedius)
- Abdominals (rectus abdominis, obliquus abdominis externus and internus, transversus abdominis)
- **Sartorius**
- Latissimus dorsi
- Tensor fascia lata
- Erector spinae

Hints for Various Age Levels

- **K-2**: Perform One-Foot Lift, perform March, and introduce Static Leg Lift 1.
- **3-5**: Add Static Leg Lift 2. With the time allotments for physical education classes, there is likely not enough time to progress to the dynamic movements, although there are many students of this age who could perform them.
- **6-12**: All the seated balances are appropriate. Keep in mind the wide range of fitness of these students. Be sure to present the exercises in a progression, and emphasize practicing at the level of capability. Build strength so that the exercises can be practiced with correct form to prevent strain.

Assessment

The assessment forms for these exercises appear as full-size forms for easy printing on the bound-in CD-ROM at the back of this book.

One-Foot Lift

Instructions

1. Starting position: Sit correctly on the ball with abdominal muscles engaged (see figure 5.2*a* on page 41).
2. Lift one foot (see figure 7.2).
3. Hold for a count of 5 to 10.
4. Replace foot on floor.
5. Repeat with other foot.

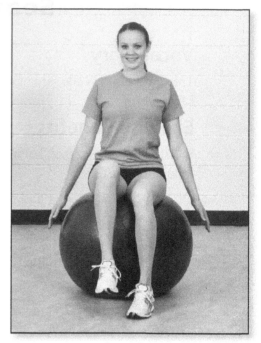

Figure 7.2 One-foot lift.

March

Instructions

1. Starting position: Sit correctly on the ball (see figure 5.2*a* on page 41).
2. March with feet in place, using quadriceps to lift feet.
3. Start with low steps, and gradually lift feet higher (see figure 7.3).

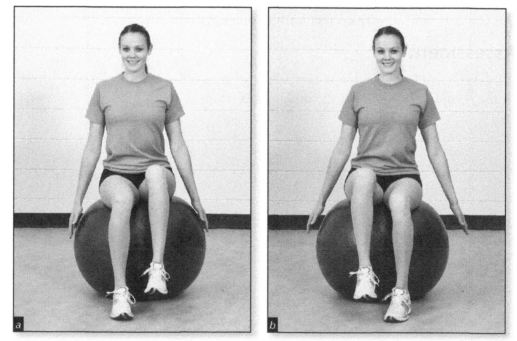

Figure 7.3 March.

Static Leg Lift 1

Instructions

1. Lift one foot, and extend leg straight in front of hip (or as high as you are comfortable doing).
2. Hold steady for a count of 5, gradually increasing the count on subsequent tries.
3. Repeat with other leg (see figure 7.4).

Variations

See Static Leg Lift 2.

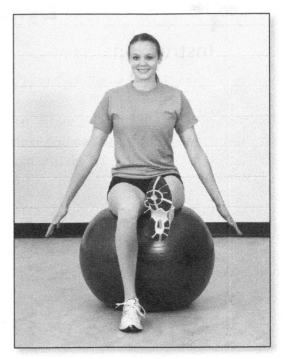

Figure 7.4 Static Leg Lift 1.

Static Leg Lift 2

Instructions

1. Starting position: Sit correctly on the ball (see figure 5.2*a* on page 41).
2. Lift one leg straight in front.
3. From the extended leg position, move the leg away from the midline toward the side.
4. Keep leg straight, and lift hip high.
5. Repeat with other leg (see figure 7.5).

Variations

See Static Leg Lift 1.

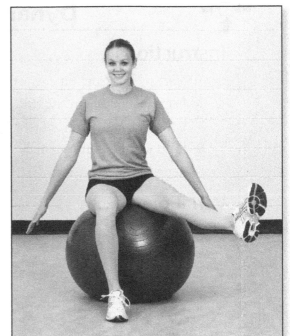

Figure 7.5 Static Leg Lift 2.

Dynamic March 1

Instructions

1. Starting position: Sit correctly on the ball (see figure 5.2*a* on page 41).
2. Begin bouncing on the ball.
3. Pick up one foot and replace, then repeat with other foot. March (see figure 7.6).

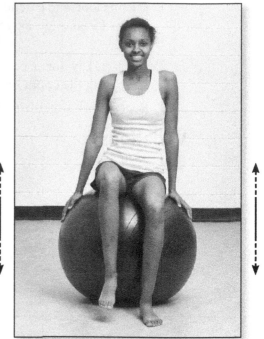

Figure 7.6 Dynamic March.

Dynamic Leg Lift 1

Instructions

1. Starting position: Sit correctly on the ball (see figure 5.2*a* on page 41).
2. Begin bouncing on the ball.
3. Lift leg straight in front (see figure 7.7*a*).
4. Hold leg and continue to bounce.
5. Repeat with other leg.

Variations

See Dynamic Leg Lift 2.

Instructions

1. Starting position: Sit correctly on the ball (see figure 5.2*a* on page 41).
2. Begin bouncing.
3. Lift leg straight in front, and then move leg away from midline.
4. Repeat with other leg.
5. These versions will challenge anyone (see figures 7.7*b*)!

Variations

See Dynamic Leg Lift 1.

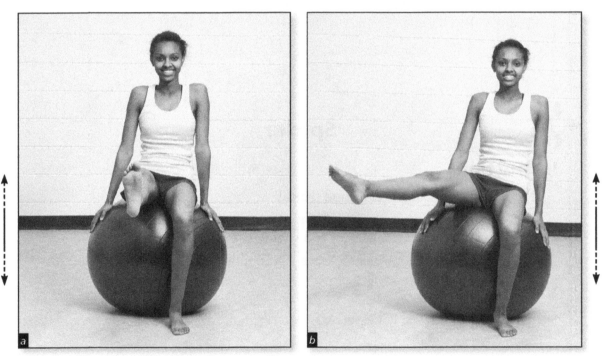

Figure 7.7 *(a)* Dynamic Leg Lift 1; *(b)* Dynamic Leg Lift 2.

Prone Balance Exercises

Vocabulary

The vocabulary is the same for all the balance exercises and should be reinforced in each lesson.

Exercise Benefits

Benefits of these prone balance exercises include the following:

- Each of these balances strengthens the torso (core muscles) and will provide support and balance in the upright body position.

- During these exercises, it will be obvious which students have a weak core. They will rest more frequently and need more encouragement to keep trying.

Hints for Various Age Levels

- **K-2:** Introduce only the first four exercises (Foot Lift, March, Static Leg Lift 1, and Static Leg Lift 2) during the first experience with these exercises.
- **3-5:** Quickly review positions for the first four exercises then add Dynamic March, Dynamic Foot Lift, Dynamic Leg Lift 1, and Dynamic Leg Lift 2.
- **6-12:** Use as a preliminary activity before strength exercises (see chapter 9, "Muscular Strength Exercises"). Note any students who seem especially weak.

Assessment

The assessment forms for these exercises appear as full-size forms for easy printing on the bound-in CD-ROM at the back of this book.

Spider

Instructions

1. Starting position: Kneel behind the ball.
2. Place stomach on the ball, and place hands on the floor in front of the ball while keeping feet on the floor and straightening knees.
3. This position is a four-point balance, not counting the stomach (see figure 7.8).

Variations

See Three, Two, and One Point Balances described on pages 75-79.

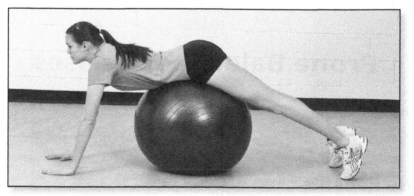

Figure 7.8 Spider.

Three-Point Balances

Instructions

1. Starting position: Get into the four-point balance you achieved in Spider.
2. Lift one hand from the floor, and stretch arm forward straight ahead of the shoulder (see figure 7.9a).
3. Hold this three-point balance for a count of 5 to 10.
4. Stress "tight" muscles and a steady position, like a statue.
5. Replace hand on floor.
6. Repeat with other hand.
7. Lift one leg off floor, and hold at hip level for 5 to 10 seconds (see figure 7.9b). Replace foot on floor.
8. Repeat with other leg.
9. Rest. Because some people have difficulty remaining prone on the ball because of pressure on the abdomen, have these people roll back to knees behind the ball and rest for 10 seconds. Take the opportunity to point out good form or to reinforce the statue idea.
10. Return to the starting position: Spider.

Variations

See Two-Point Balances described on pages 76 and 78.

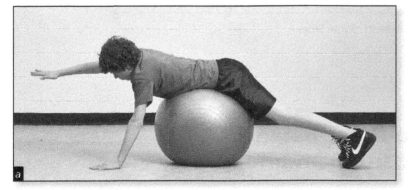

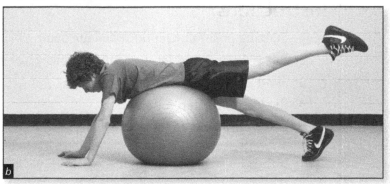

Figure 7.9 Three-Point Balances: *(a)* one arm; *(b)* one leg.

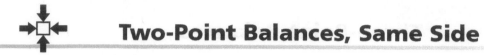

Two-Point Balances, Same Side

Instructions

1. Starting position: Get into the four-point balance you achieved in Spider.
2. Lift left arm and left leg simultaneously (see figure 7.10).
3. Hold for a count of 5 to 10.
4. Replace hand and foot to the floor.
5. Repeat actions with other arm and leg.
6. Rest.

Variations

See Two-Point Balances, Opposite Arm and Leg on this page.

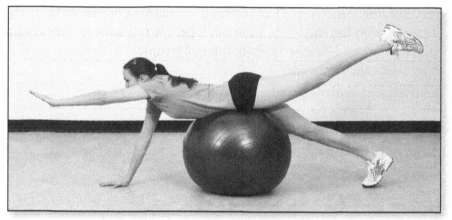

Figure 7.10   Two-Point Balances, Same Side.

Two-Point Balances, Opposite Arm and Leg

Instructions

1. Starting position: Get into the four-point balance you achieved in Spider.
2. Lift right arm and left leg simultaneously (see figure 7.11).
3. Hold for a count of 5 to 10.
4. Replace hand and foot on floor.
5. Repeat previous actions with left arm and right leg. Notice these last two steps are considerably harder to maintain in a steady manner. Muscles will probably quiver for many students at first.
6. Rest.

Variations

See Two-Point Balances, Same Side on page 76.

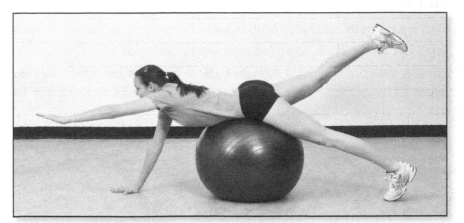

Figure 7.11 Two-Point Balance: Opposite Arm and Leg.

Superman/Wonder Woman

Instructions

1. Starting position: Get into the four-point balance you achieved in Spider.
2. With hands on floor, rock weight toward feet.
3. Lift both hands from floor, and extend arms forward (see figure 7.12). This is a Superman or Wonder Woman position with the arms stretched to sides at shoulder level (airplane position) or a combination of one arm ahead and one arm to the side. Use back extensors (muscles of the lower back) to anchor the body.
4. Return to starting position.
5. Rest.

Variations

This exercise becomes "The Airplane" when arms are held straight to the side.

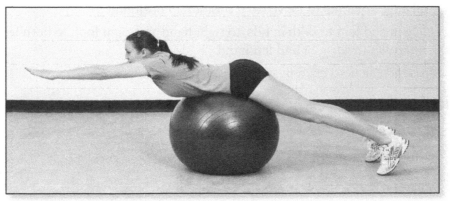

Figure 7.12 Superman/Wonder Woman.

Two-Hand Balance

Instructions

1. Starting position: Get into the four-point balance you achieved in Spider.
2. With feet on the floor, rock and shift weight to hands.
3. Lift legs off floor and hold straight back at hip level for 5 to 10 seconds (see figure 7.13).
4. Return feet to floor.
5. Rest.

Variations

See Superman/Wonder Woman on page 77.

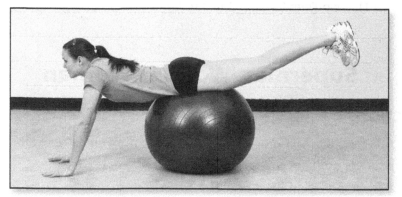

Figure 7.13   Two-Hand Balance.

Weight Transfer and Balance (Dynamic Balance)

Instructions

1. Starting position: Get into the four-point balance you achieved in Spider.
2. Challenge students to move from position to position.
3. Left arm and foot to both hands, to right hand and right foot, to both feet, and then return to left foot and left hand.
4. Momentarily hold each position.

Variations

Reverse the direction of the weight transfer.

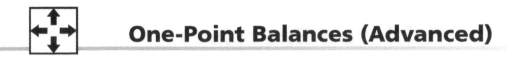

One-Point Balances (Advanced)

Instructions

1. Starting position: Get into the four-point balance you achieved in Spider.
2. Challenge students to balance with only one body part touching the floor (see figure 7.14, *a* and *b*).

Variations

See if participants can do weight transfer (similar to Weight Transfer and Balance on page 78) and keep balanced. Right foot, left foot, left hand, right hand. Reverse direction.

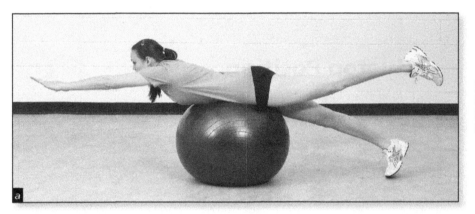

Figure 7.14 One-Point Balances: *(a)* right foot or left foot; *(b)* right hand or left hand.

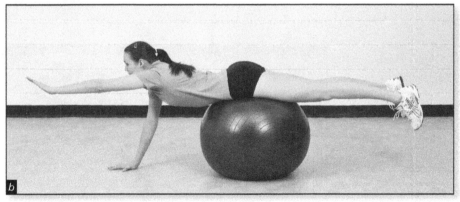

Tabletop Exercises

Vocabulary

The vocabulary is the same for all the balance exercises and should be reinforced in each lesson.

Assessment

The assessment forms for these exercises appear as full-size forms for easy printing on the bound-in CD-ROM at the back of this book.

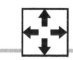

Tabletop Position

Before continuing, assess to see if the student or client can keep

- feet shoulder-width apart (or closer),
- shoulder blades on the ball, and
- hips lifted so that there is a straight line from shoulders to knees (see figure 7.15).

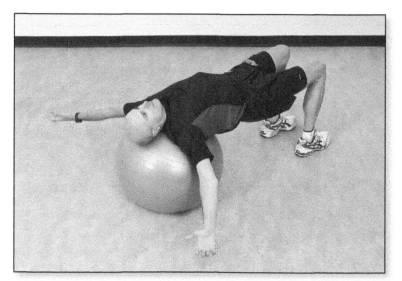

Figure 7.15 Correct Tabletop position.

Tabletop March

Instructions

1. Starting position: Get into Tabletop position (see figure 7.15).
2. Lift one foot off floor (contract abs and use quads) and replace. Repeat with other foot.
3. Attempt to shift weight back and forth as if walking. Do not let hips sag (see figure 7.16).
4. *Note:* At first only a few steps will be possible before starting to wobble.

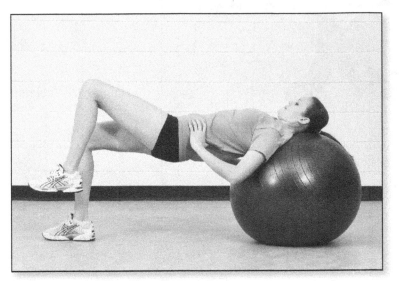

Figure 7.16 Tabletop March.

Exercise Benefits

- Instability of the ball engages muscles of the back (**erector spinae**), abdomen, and buttocks (**gluteus**) as well as the hamstrings (biceps femoris and semitendinosus).
- The foot lift is performed by the quadriceps and hip flexors.

Hints for Various Age Levels

- **K-2**: Those students who can hold the Tabletop position can try small foot lifts. Most students will have a hard time keeping their hips lifted.
- **3-5**: Most students can perform the march. It will be a challenge for some.
- **6-12**: These students should work on increasing the number of steps (marches) they can perform. They should stop when their form deteriorates.

Tabletop Sway

Instructions

1. Starting position: Get into Tabletop position (see figure 7.15).
2. With shoulders, roll ball away from the midline to one side.
3. As the torso muscles engage and you feel almost ready to fall, roll (pull with torso) the ball back to midline (see figure 7.17). Repeat on other side.
4. As torso gets stronger, increase movement away from midline.

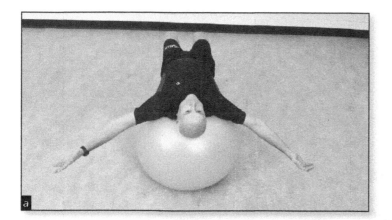

Figure 7.17 Tabletop Sway.

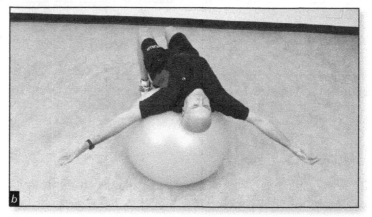

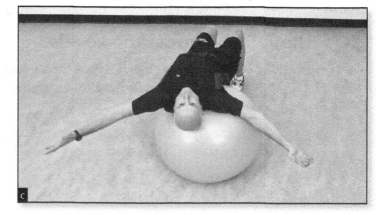

Exercise Benefits

An incredible workout for the abdominals, especially the obliques, as well as challenging the back, buttocks, and hamstrings.

Hints for Various Age Levels

- **K-2**: Too difficult for most K-2 students.
- **3-5**: Introduce this exercise to people with strong torso muscles. Other people can work on the Tabletop position or the Tabletop March.
- **6-12**: This age level will enjoy the challenge. Ask them to start small and to know their limits. They should not fall each time they attempt the sway, but rather learn to know when they are almost ready to fall and to pull back to midline.

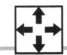

One-Leg Tabletop

Instructions

1. Starting position: Get into Tabletop position (see figure 7.15).
2. Lift one foot from floor, and extend leg straight in line with hip.
3. Hold for as long as possible, then replace foot on floor (see figure 7.18). Repeat with other foot.

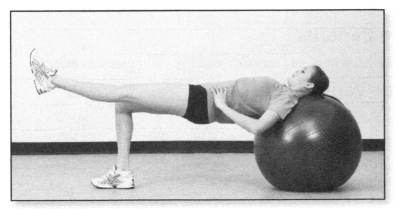

Figure 7.18   One-Leg Tabletop.

Exercise Benefits

Abdominals, back muscles, buttocks, and legs as in previous exercise.

Hints for Various Age Levels

- **K-2**: Too difficult for most K-2 students.
- **3-5**: Encourage students to lift the leg momentarily and then set it down. Repeat on other side and rest. This is a strenuous exercise. They can do another set of one rep on each side, if they rest.
- **6-12**: This age level can work on increasing the time they hold each repetition or can do two or more repetitions on each side before resting.

Advanced One-Leg Tabletop

Instructions

1. Starting position: Get into Tabletop position (see figure 7.15).
2. Lift one foot from floor, and extend leg straight in line with hip.
3. Move leg away from midline to side, keeping leg straight and lifted (see figure 7.19).
4. Bring back to midline. Repeat with other leg.

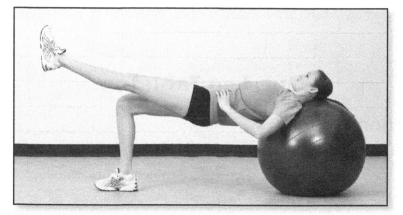

Figure 7.19   Advanced One-Leg Tabletop.

Exercise Benefits

Abdominals, back muscles, buttocks, and legs as in previous exercise.

Hints for Various Age Levels

- **K-2**: Too difficult for most K-2 students.
- **3-5**: Too difficult for most 3-5 students.
- **6-12**: Introduce this exercise after your group can hold One-Leg Tabletop for 5 to 10 seconds.

Other Balance Exercises

The remaining balances are advanced. The Side-Lying Balance builds on the basic position from chapter 5 and has both legs extended to challenge balance. Hands and Knees Balance and Knee Balance are for advanced students and should be spotted for safety.

Side-Lying Balance

Vocabulary

The vocabulary is the same for all the balance exercises and should be reinforced in each lesson.

Instructions

1. Starting position: Kneel on the floor with the ball at the side, hand on the ball.
2. Lean hip and lay side of torso on the ball, sliding the hand and arm over the ball (see figure 7.20*a* on this page).
3. Straighten top leg until it extends straight from hip.
4. With hand of bottom arm on floor, straighten lower leg and foot to meet upper foot (see 7.20*b*). Feet can be one behind the other (on the floor) or stacked on top of one another (see 7.20*c*).
5. Keep body perpendicular to the floor. This will force engagement of all muscles in the torso.
6. Repeat on other side.

(continued)

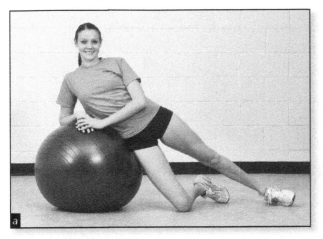
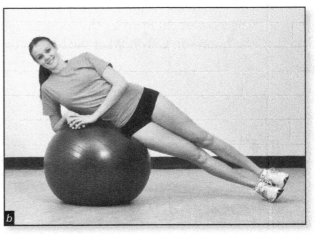
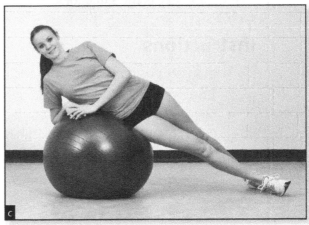

Figure 7.20 Side-Lying Balance.

Exercise Benefits

This exercise strengthens core muscles, both the front and back of the torso and especially the oblique muscles.

Variations

1. **Advanced action:** For those who can maintain the balance with steadiness and little wobble, have them take the hand off the floor and place it on the ball. At first there will be a bit of wobble. Next, take the hand and arm off the ball and extend the arm in a straight line with the body. The upper arm may also be extended overhead with hands meeting. Students hold this position for 5 seconds, gradually extending the time balanced. This balance is essential for exercises in the strength chapter.

2. **Reflection:** Have students note if one side is easier or harder than the other. Explain that this is normal, although they will want to strengthen the weaker side. Next time, have them start on the more difficult side, then switch sides; finally, repeat the balance on the weaker side for more practice.

Hints for Various Age Levels

This an advanced balance and best suits students or clients of middle school age or older.

Assessment

The assessment form for this exercise appears as a full-size form for easy printing on the bound-in CD-ROM at the back of this book.

Hands and Knees Balance

Vocabulary

The vocabulary is the same for all the balance exercises and should be reinforced in each lesson.

Instructions

1. Starting position: Stand with the ball in front of feet, both hands on the ball.
2. Bring one knee up and place on the ball.
3. Place weight on hands and knee while attempting to place other knee on ball (see figure 7.21).
4. The challenge is to see how long you can balance.

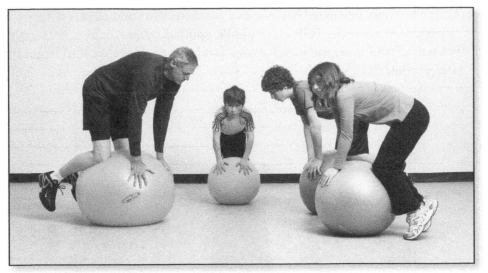

Figure 7.21 Hands and Knees Balance.

Exercise Benefits

This exercise is a full body balance challenge.

Variations

See Knee Balance on this page.

Hints for Various Age Levels

Appropriate for middle school and older.

Assessment

The assessment form for this exercise appears as a full-size form for easy printing on the bound-in CD-ROM at the back of this book.

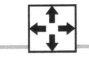

Knee Balance

Vocabulary

The vocabulary is the same for all the balance exercises and should be reinforced in each lesson.

Instructions

1. Starting position: Stand behind the ball with hands on the ball.
2. Move to the Hands and Knees Balance as described in the previous exercise.
3. Shift weight to knees and shins while raising upper body toward upright.
4. Remove one hand from the ball and then the second (see figure 7.22).

(continued)

5. *Note:* This is an advanced balance and is for students and clients who are very experienced with the ball. It should be spotted by one or two persons until the participant is secure in achieving this balance. It is easiest to begin on an underinflated (squishy) ball.

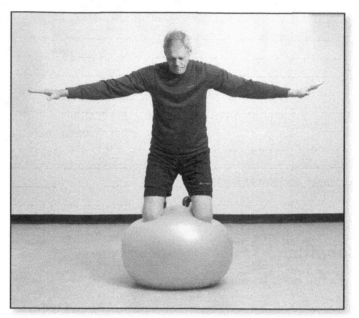

Figure 7.22   Knee Balance.

Exercise Benefits

This exercise is a full body balance challenge.

Hints for Various Age Levels

Only for clients or students who are high school age or older.

Assessment

The assessment form for this exercise appears as a full-size form for easy printing on the bound-in CD-ROM at the back of this book.

eight

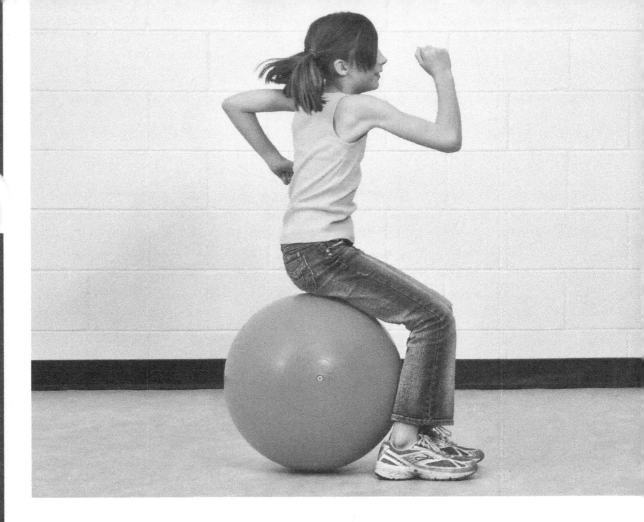

Cardiorespiratory Fitness Exercises

Cardiorespiratory fitness is the health of the heart (cardio) and lungs (respiratory). Exercise that causes the heart to beat faster strengthens the heart muscle. A healthy, strong heart and circulatory system means that the blood (which carries oxygen to the muscles) is pumped more efficiently and effectively. Because oxygen use is increased during exercise, it is often referred to as **aerobic exercise**.

Raising the heart rate and breathing faster by simply bouncing on an exercise ball are two major signs of cardiorespiratory exercise, and they are also signs that the exercise ball is an excellent piece of equipment to obtain and maintain aerobic health. An exercise ball provides a low-impact, gentle, comfortable cardiorespiratory workout while challenging balance and strengthening the core muscles, as we discussed in the previous two chapters. By adding arm movements, feet movements, and combinations of the two to ball bouncing, you can add both intensity and variety to create your cardiorespiratory workout. The exercises in this chapter describe some of the many exercise variations possible on the exercise ball.

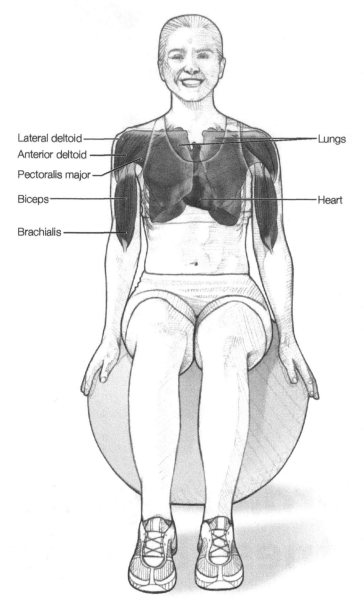

Lateral deltoid

Anterior deltoid

Pectoralis major

Biceps

Brachialis

Lungs

Heart

Muscles and organs of upper torso and upper arm muscles.

Basic Bounce

Instructions

1. Starting position: Sit on the center of the ball, not the front. You want the bounce to go straight down through the center of the ball.

2. Sit tall in good posture. Do not slump or round the back. Your vertebrae should be stacked like blocks.

3. Engage your abdominal muscles by sucking in the belly button. Some people envision this better by thinking of scooping the belly.

4. Initially the hands should be at the sides of the ball, touching lightly (see figure 8.1*a*). With practice the hands can be held away from the ball or on the thighs (see figure 8.1*b*). Beginners will want to start with small, controlled bounces, taking care to keep feet on the floor. Often exuberant students will jump as they bounce, not realizing that the rebound of the ball could send them or the ball flying.

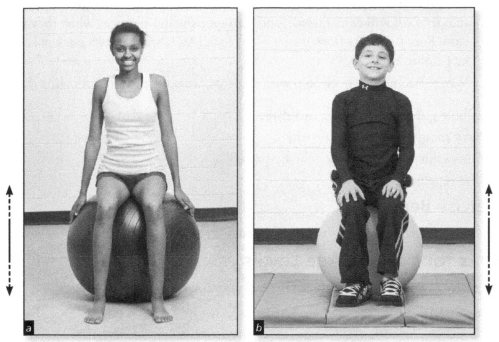

Figure 8.1   Basic Bounce: *(a)* hands at the sides of the ball; *(b)* hands on thighs.

Exercise Benefits

This exercise raises the heart rate while challenging balance and strengthening the torso.

Variations

See Check Stop on page 92.

Hints for Various Age Levels

Appropriate for all ages.

Assessment

The assessment form for this exercise appears as a full-size form for easy printing on the bound-in CD-ROM at the back of this book.

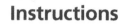

Check Stop

Instructions

1. Starting position: Sit correctly on the ball (see figure 5.2a on page 41).

2. It is important to practice how to stop bouncing, especially with elementary-age students, so participants will understand that they are in control. Explain that the ball will continue to bounce in ever smaller bounces when they try to stop. *Keep feet on the floor in a wide stance, and hold arms out from sides for balance* (see figure 8.2).

3. When practicing Check Stop with students, we bounce to the following rhyme:

Bubble gum, bubble gum, in a dish.

How many pieces do you wish?

One, (pause), two, (pause), three, (pause),

POP! (pause) STOP!

Exercise Benefits

This exercise promotes safe usage of the exercise ball.

Hints for Various Age Levels

Especially important for young users (K-2) and novice users.

Assessment

The assessment form for this exercise appears as a full-size form for easy printing on the bound-in CD-ROM at the back of this book.

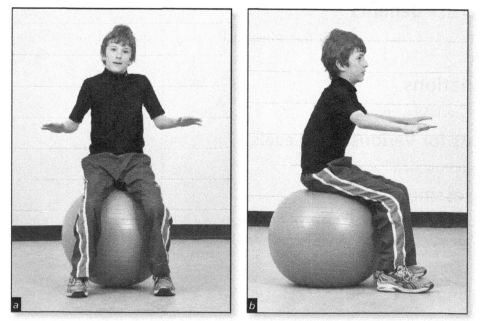

Figure 8.2 *(a)* Check Stop from front; *(b)* Check Stop from side.

Arm Exercises

This section describes a few of the many arm movements that participants can perform on the ball. Initially the arms are practiced with plain bouncing and feet kept on the floor. Moving the arms can cause a slight loss of balance for novice users of the exercise ball.

Exercise Benefits

This exercise raises the heart rate by adding body parts (arms) to the movement and promotes safe usage of the exercise ball by introducing one additional variable at a time.

Hints for Various Age Levels

Especially important for young users (K-2) and novice users.

Assessment

The assessment forms for these exercises appear as full-size forms for easy printing on the bound-in CD-ROM at the back of this book.

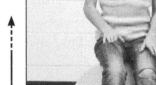

Pat

Instructions

1. Starting position: Sit correctly on the ball (see figure 5.2a on page 41).

2. Lightly pat the thighs in rhythm with the bouncing (see figure 8.3).

3. Keep rhythm with the bounce of the ball. Movement of the arms increases the amplitude of the bounce.

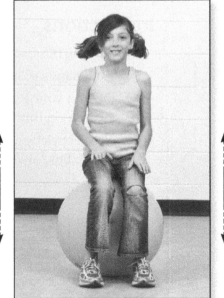

Figure 8.3 Pat and bounce.

Push

Instructions

1. Starting position: Sit correctly on the ball (see figure 5.2a on page 41).

2. With hands by the sides, push hands down and lift up.

3. Start with small pushes of the air beside the ball, and gradually increase (see figure 8.4).

4. The lifting and pushing increase the size of the bounce and raise the heart rate.

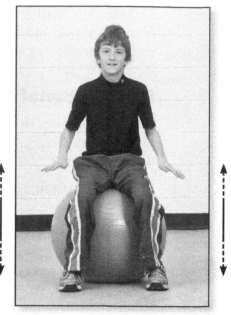

Figure 8.4 Push and lift.

Windshield Washing

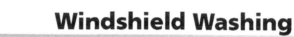

Instructions

1. Starting position: Sit correctly on the ball (see figure 5.2a on page 41).

2. Hold hands in front of body as if there were a window in front of you.

3. Pretend your hands are windshield wipers, and wipe the window back and forth in rhythm with the bounce (see figure 8.5).

4. *Note:* For elementary-age students or preschoolers, it is fun to sing "The Wheels on the Bus," making all the motions while bouncing. Now that is brainwork!

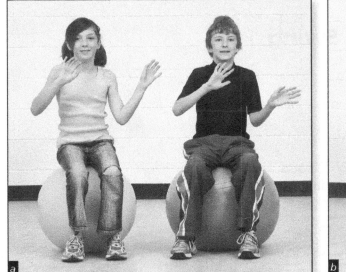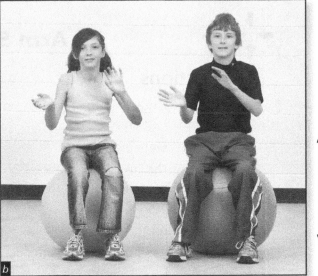

Figure 8.5 Windshield Washing.

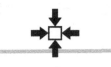

Rainbow Arms

Instructions

1. Rainbow Arms is a larger sweep of the hands similar to Windshield Washing.

2. Starting position: Sit correctly on the ball (see figure 5.2a on page 41).

3. Hold hands in front of the body, and make a large inverted-U shape, with the hands extending upward, arching, and coming down.

4. This raising of the hands and arms will increase the amplitude of the bounce and almost lift you off the ball (see figure 8.6).

5. Be sure to remind your group to use control while practicing.

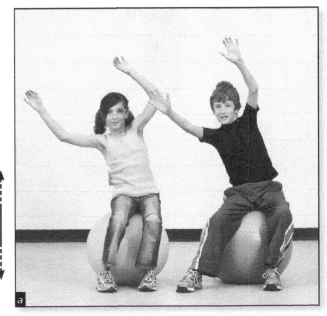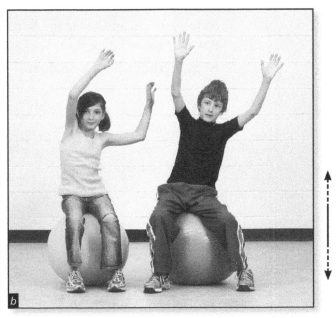

Figure 8.6 Rainbow arms.

Arm Swing 1

Instructions

1. Starting position: Sit correctly on the ball (see figure 5.2a on page 41).
2. Begin bouncing.
3. Swing the arms simultaneously forward and back along the sides of the body and the ball (see figure 8.7).
4. Keep rhythm with the bounce.
5. The arm swing can rise to shoulder level in front.

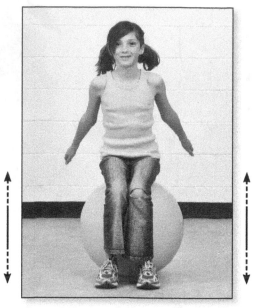

Figure 8.7 Arm Swing 1.

Arm Swing 2

Instructions

1. Starting position: Sit correctly on the ball (see figure 5.2a on page 41).
2. Begin bouncing.
3. Swing arms in an alternating fashion, as if walking (see figure 8.8).
4. Keep rhythm with the bounce.

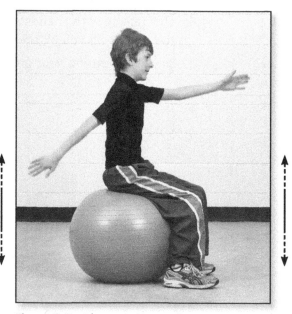

Figure 8.8 Alternate arm swing.

Instructions

1. Starting position: Sit correctly on the ball (see figure 5.2a on page 41).

2. Begin bouncing.

3. Hold arms bent in a right angle as if running.

4. Swing arms alternately back and forth as if running (see figure 8.9).

5. Smaller swings will result in lower bounces, and conversely, larger swings result in larger bounces.

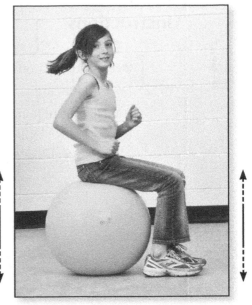

Figure 8.9 Runner Arms.

Feet Exercises

Moving the feet will increase the heart rate even more. These exercises start with one foot moving at a time to help maintain balance. Jumping (both feet off the floor at once) is introduced once participants are competent and confident.

Exercise Benefits

This exercise increases heart rate by using the large muscles of the legs.

Hints for Various Age Levels

Novice users should master the Dynamic March 2 and Heel and Toe Touches before moving to the jumping exercises.

Assessment

The assessment forms for these exercises appear as full-size forms for easy printing on the bound-in CD-ROM at the back of this book.

Dynamic March 2

Instructions

1. Starting position: Sit correctly on the ball (see figure 5.2*a* on page 41).
2. Begin bouncing.
3. Alternately lift one foot at a time and replace it (see figure 8.10).
4. This will feel like walking or marching in place.

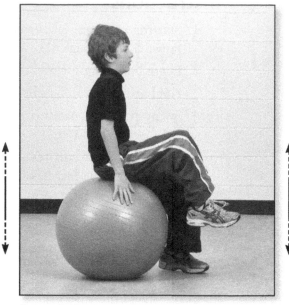

Figure 8.10   Dynamic March.

Heel Touches

Instructions

1. Starting position: Sit correctly on the ball (see figure 5.2*a* on page 41).
2. Begin bouncing.
3. Alternately lift one foot at a time, and touch the heel to the floor about 12 inches (30 cm) in front of the ball and then replace it.
4. This is a two-count move, and one foot always remains on the ground (see figure 8.11).
5. *Note:* With more practice it can become Cossack by making it one count per foot.

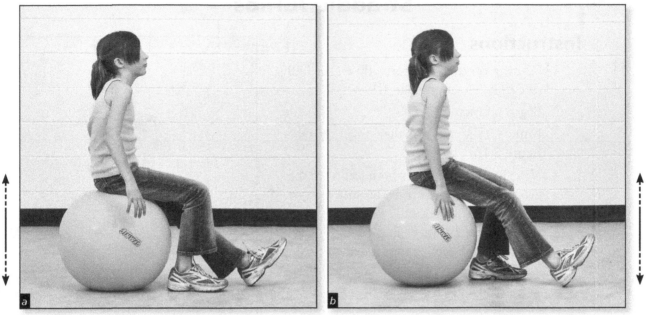

Figure 8.11 Heel Touches.

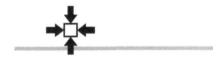

Toe Touches

Instructions

1. Starting position: Sit correctly on the ball (see figure 5.2*a* on page 41).

2. Begin bouncing.

3. Alternately lift one foot at a time, and touch the toe about 12 inches (30 cm) to the side (see figure 8.12).

4. This also is a two-count move: toe touch, count one; replace foot to original place, count two.

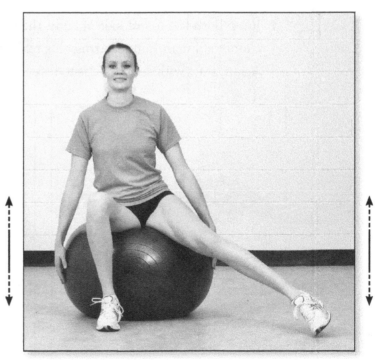

Figure 8.12 Toe Touches.

Straddle Jumps

Instructions

1. Starting position: Sit correctly on the ball (see figure 5.2a on page 41).
2. Begin bouncing.
3. Jump feet apart and then together (see figure 8.13).
4. *Note:* Jumping removes both feet from the ground at the same time. Be sure to start with small bounces and small jumps until sure of your balance. Engage abdominal muscles, and keep spine straight.

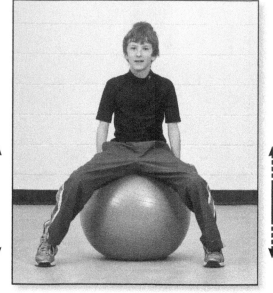

Figure 8.13   Straddle Jumps.

Skier

Instructions

1. Starting position: Sit correctly on the ball (see figure 5.2a on page 41).
2. Begin bouncing.
3. Jump both feet to one side of body, then jump feet to other side.
4. Combined with Runner Arms, this really mimics skiing (see figure 8.14).
5. Again, start with small jumps to test your dynamic balance.

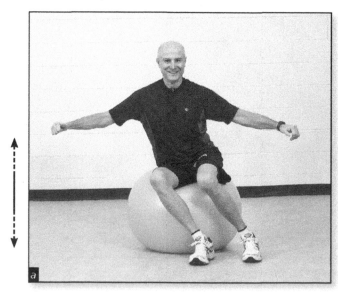 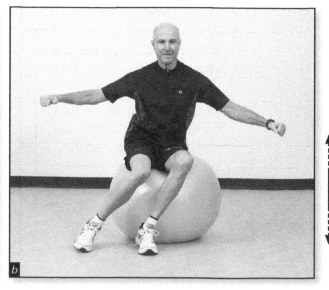

Figure 8.14   Skier.

Instructions

1. Starting position: Sit correctly on the ball (see figure 5.2*a* on page 41).

2. Begin bouncing.

3. Do heel touches, alternating feet without replacing feet in the starting stance (see figure 8.15).

4. This becomes a jump, then, because both feet are off the floor at the same time.

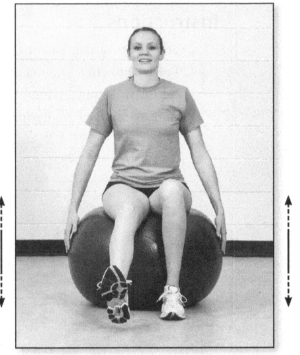

Figure 8.15 Cossack.

Combined Arms and Feet Exercises

For beginning users of the ball, it is best to practice arms alone first, as this requires less of a balance challenge. Second, foot moves are practiced solo. This allows the exerciser to concentrate on the feet and use the arms to maintain balance. In this section, we combine arms and feet for an even more vigorous workout.

Exercise Benefits

Using both arms and legs while bouncing raises the heart rate even higher and challenges balance even more.

Hints for Various Age Levels

Caution all users to remember safety, especially novice users. The joy of bouncing can result in over exuberant movement that can cause a fall.

Assessment

The assessment forms for these exercises appear as full-size forms for easy printing on the bound-in CD-ROM at the back of this book.

March With Arm Swing

Instructions

1. Starting position: Sit correctly on the ball (see figure 8.16a).
2. Begin bouncing, and march feet.
3. Add Arm Swing 1 (simultaneous arm swing) (see figure 8.16b).
4. Add Arm Swing 2 (alternate arm swing) (see figure 8.16c).

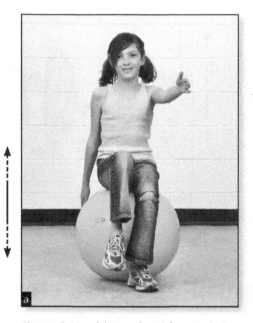

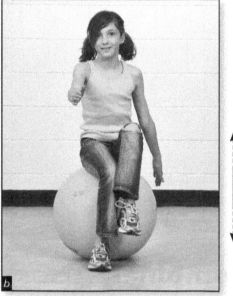

Figure 8.16 *(a)* March With Arm Swing starting position; *(b)* March With Arm Swing 1; *(c)* March With Arm Swing 2.

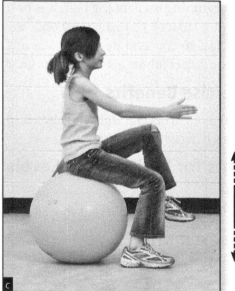

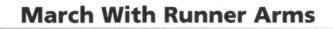

March With Runner Arms

Instructions

1. Starting position: Sit correctly on the ball (see figure 5.2*a* on page 41).

2. Bounce with feet marching.

3. Add Runner Arms (see figure 8.17). It will feel as if you are almost moving down the street.

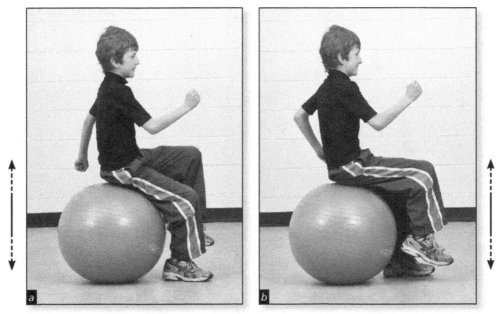

Figure 8.17   March With Runner Arms.

Skier With Runner Arms

Instructions

1. Starting position: Sit correctly on the ball (see figure 5.2*a* on page 41).
2. Begin bouncing, and hold Runner Arms.
3. As you begin the Skier jump, move both hands toward the opposite side of body.
4. Alternate feet and arms in opposition (see figure 8.18).
5. You will feel as if you are skiing. This is excellent practice for the real thing.

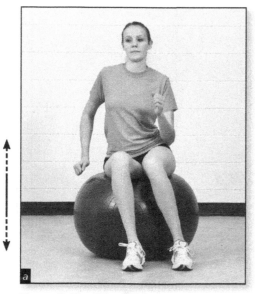
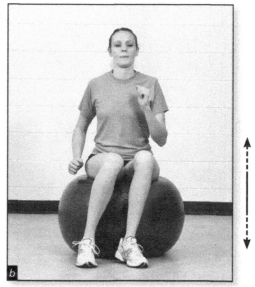

Figure 8.18   Skier With Runner Arms.

Jumping Jacks

Instructions

1. Starting position: Sit correctly on the ball (see figure 5.2*a* on page 41).
2. This exercise combines a straddle jump with jumping jack arms.
3. Begin bouncing, and raise arms to the side while doing a straddle jump.
4. The arms can stop at shoulder height for a half jack (see figure 8.19*a*) or overhead for a full jack (see figure 8.19*b*).

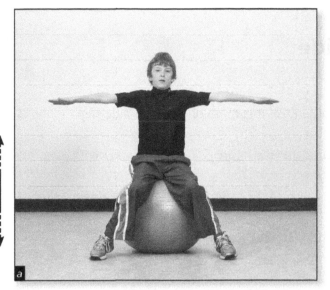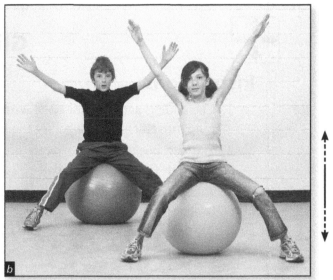

Figure 8.19 Jumping Jacks: *(a)* half jack; *(b)* full jack.

Cossack With Arms Crossed

Instructions

1. Starting position: Sit correctly on the ball (see figure 5.2*a* on page 41).

2. Begin bouncing, and do heel touches alternating 1-2-1-2.

3. As you become comfortable with Cossack feet, lift arms away from sides and cross arms over chest (see figure 8.20).

4. By removing the arms from a position that assists balance, you increase the challenge to your core muscles.

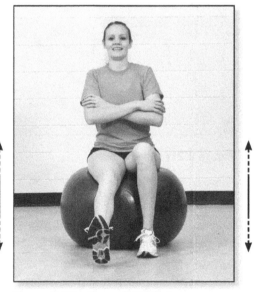

Figure 8.20 Cossack With Arms Crossed.

Instructions

1. The glide is actually not done with a bounce. It is more of a side-to-side stepping movement with a roll of the ball.

2. Starting position: Sit correctly on the ball (see figure 5.2a on page 41) with hands at the sides of the ball.

3. Take a small step to one side, and then bring the other foot and touch it next to the stepping foot.

4. Without putting weight on the second foot, take a step to the other side.

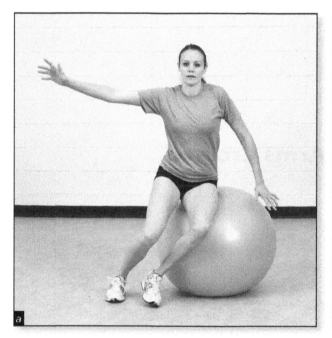

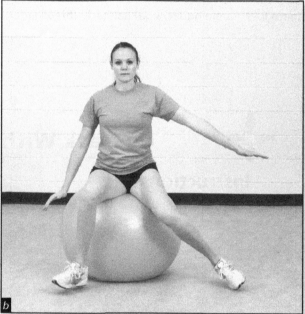

Figure 8.21 Glide.

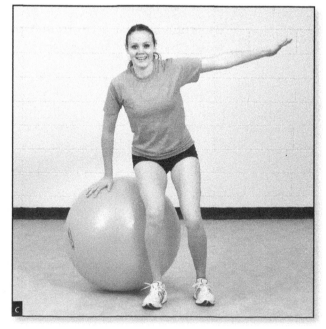

5. The arm on the stepping side will almost automatically lift upward for balance, and the ball will begin to roll side to side.

6. As you get more adept at this move, add a pause as you reach the top of your sideways movement before you transfer your weight to the other side (see figure 8.21). It should feel like a swing gliding.

7. The glide is a real workout for the quadriceps when you are able to almost stand up at the pause.

nine

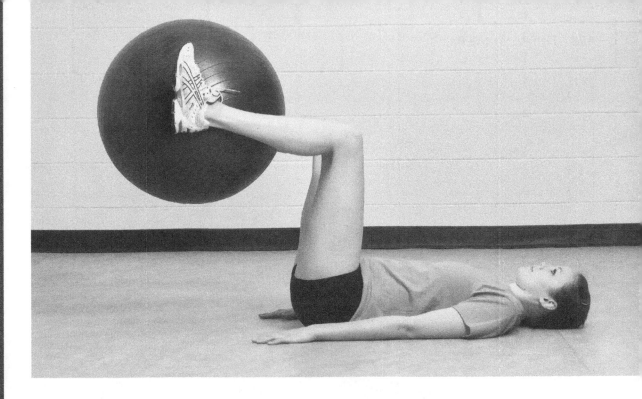

Muscular Strength Exercises

M uscular **strength** can be developed through moving the body's muscles against **resistance**. Resistance can be provided by a person's own weight, by lifting a weight, or by resistance bands and tubes. Just moving a muscle will maintain the strength it has. Conversely, not moving a muscle will result in **atrophy**, or weaker muscles. To make a muscle stronger, the muscle must lift, hold, pull, or push a weight heavier than normal. This is the principle of **overload**. Overload can also be provided by increasing the frequency, intensity, or duration (length of **time**) of the exercise.

Intensity refers to how difficult an exercise is. Intensity in strength workouts can be changed by doing an exercise very slowly or very quickly. It can also be made harder by gradually increasing the amount of weight. At the same weight, intensity can also be varied by decreasing the rest period between sets of one exercise or between different exercises.

In this chapter, we present exercises that are primarily muscular strength activities. As with all exercise ball activities, a large component of balance accompanies each of these exercises. That is what makes ball exercises so beneficial—the necessary engagement of ancillary muscles results in dynamic, authentic strength *and* balance.

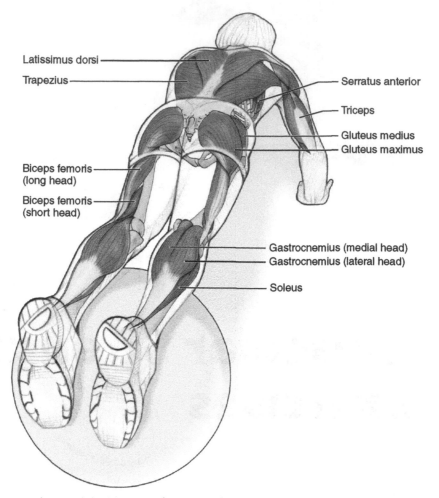

Latissimus dorsi

Trapezius

Serratus anterior

Triceps

Gluteus medius
Gluteus maximus

Biceps femoris
(long head)

Biceps femoris
(short head)

Gastrocnemius (medial head)
Gastrocnemius (lateral head)

Soleus

Muscles used during muscular strength exercises. The engagement of these muscles results in dynamic, authentic strength and balance.

All muscular strength workouts consist of a specific number of **repetitions**, or **reps**. Repetitions refer to the number of times an exercise is repeated before stopping to rest. A number of repetitions done sequentially without a rest is called a **set**. Therefore, 8 repetitions done twice with a period of rest in between each set of 8 are referred to as 2 sets of 8 repetitions rather than 16 repetitions. It is important to understand repetitions and sets because they are utilized in various ways to design workouts that focus on building muscle, maintaining muscle, or increasing muscle endurance.

To build muscle, start with a light weight and perform one set of 8 repetitions. Repeat this workout three times a week until it feels easy. Then increase the number of repetitions to 12 or 15. At this point, switch to two sets of 8 repetitions. The next step is to increase repetitions in both sets. Finally a third set can be added, or the weight can be increased. To maintain muscle once you have built muscle, work out at the level you wish to maintain. To increase muscle endurance, the workout needs to increase in duration, increasing time with each subsequent workout. As a muscle grows stronger, the number of exercise reps or sets can be increased. This is called **progression**, and it should always be done gradually.

Muscles are composed of long strings of cells called fibers. **Muscle fibers** enlarge when they perform work that is slightly heavier than usual. It's important to note that for very young students (K-2), unfit people of any age, and older adults who have not done exercise for a while, no actual weight even needs to be used, and any number of repetitions will provide a heavier load for them. You should always start with exercises that use the body's own weight as resistance. Then as a person's muscular strength increases, you can add bands, tubes, or weights of light resistance.

Muscular strength workouts should be done a minimum of two times a week, although once a week is better than not at all. The number of times per week someone completes a muscular strength workout is referred to as **frequency**. No matter what frequency is chosen, there must be one day of rest between strength workouts to allow time for muscle tissue recovery. Therefore, every other day is the maximum you should do a strength workout. Some people divide their workouts by their different muscle groups and rotate each group with every strength workout. For example, on Monday they may exercise their arms and back, and on Tuesday they may exercise their legs and abdominals. By doing this, each muscle group is resting one day.

As with all exercise types (strength, flexibility, aerobic, or balance), the improvements that result from exercise will disappear if the exercise is stopped. This **regression**, of course, occurs in all manner of skills, whether it be playing a musical instrument, solving logic problems such as sudoku, or building strength.

Each of the exercises in this chapter is grouped by the major body part that benefits from the exercise described. This does not mean this muscle is the only muscle to benefit from the exercise; it means that this muscle is the primary focus of the exercise. This is the principle of **specificity**. Each muscle needs to be targeted during exercise. Doing sit-ups will not strengthen the arms.

The easy way to remember these concepts are the acronyms **FITT** and SPORT. The FITT letters stand for

- F = frequency
- I = intensity
- T = time or duration
- T = type or component of exercise, such as balance, strength, or cardiorespiratory exercise.

The FITT concepts are the guidelines for exercising.
The SPORT letters stand for

- S = specificity
- P = progression
- O = overload
- R = regression
- T = train and maintain.

The SPORT concepts are the principles that underlie fitness development. (Virgilio 1997).

Muscle Group 1: Arms and Shoulder Girdle Exercises

The exercises in this muscle group are described from easiest to hardest (push-ups done on the ball). The exercises should be done in order because everyone likes to be successful, and it allows the students or clients to understand the progression and to work at their own level. If an exercise is too difficult, it will not be done and will not encourage commitment to an exercise program. Becoming fit will be fun if the students and clients know there is a gradual progression to improvement.

Exercise Benefits

The following exercises strengthen the arms and shoulder girdle, allowing the participant to lift or carry heavier objects more easily.

Hints for Various Age Levels

Young children (K-2) and novice exercisers should start with the Rocking Push-Up and progress as they are able. For all participants the Rocking Push-Up is a perfect place to start, and then introduce the progression.

Assessment

The assessment forms for these exercises appear as full-size forms for easy printing on the bound-in CD-ROM at the back of this book.

Rocking Push-Up

Instructions

1. Starting position: Lie prone on the ball. Place hands and feet on floor.
2. Engage abdominal muscles, arms, and shoulders as you push gently with feet (see figure 9.1*a*).
3. Bend elbows, and slowly lower the head toward the floor.
4. Touch nose lightly to the floor, and then return feet to the floor by pushing with arms (see figure 9.1*b*).
5. *Note:* Almost everyone can do this push-up because the body weight is supported by the ball.

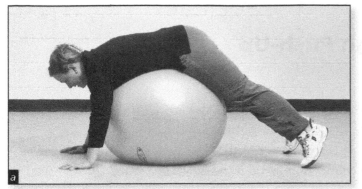

Figure 9.1 Rocking Push-Up:
(a) rocking forward; *(b)* touching
nose.

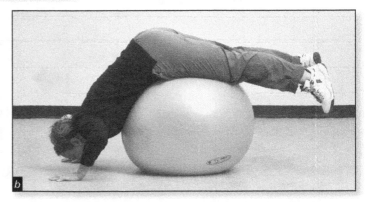

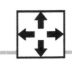

Belly Button Push-Up

Instructions

1. Starting position: Lie prone on the ball, belly button slightly forward of the center of the ball and legs together, toes touching lightly (see figure 9.2a).

2. Without rocking, bend arms and lower nose to the ground (see figure 9.2b). Be sure to engage all muscles: Do not be a limp noodle.

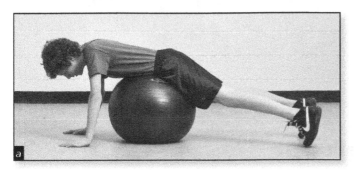

Figure 9.2 *(a)* Belly Button Push-Up starting position; *(b)* Belly Button Push-Up.

3. Push back to starting position.

4. When doing numerous repetitions, do not touch feet to ground when returning to starting position.

5. *Note:* The arms begin to take more of the body weight in this position.

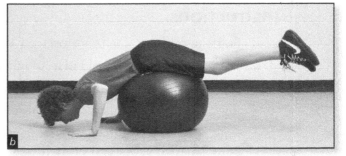

Thigh Push-Up

Instructions

1. Starting position: Lie prone on the ball. Walk hands forward until thighs are on the ball and belly button is forward of the diameter of the ball.

2. As in Belly Button Push-Up, lower nose to the floor by bending arms and engaging all muscles through contraction on both the down phase and the up phase (see figure 9.3).

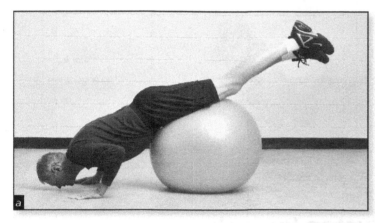

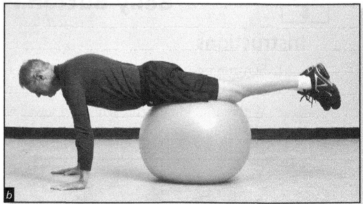

Figure 9.3 Thigh Push-Up.

Walk-Out

Instructions

1. Starting position: Lie prone on the ball.
2. Lift feet off floor and hold in a straight line with shoulders.
3. Walk hands forward, letting the ball roll (see figure 9.4).
4. Reverse the hand walk when the position becomes unstable and before falling.
5. *Note:* This exercise helps strengthen the arms and helps practice the whole-body balance necessary for more demanding progressions.

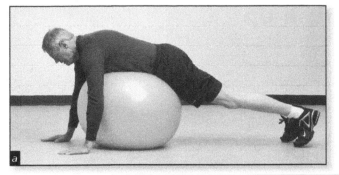

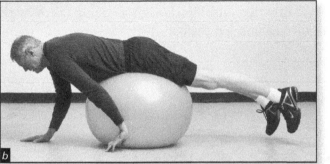

Figure 9.4   Walk-Out.

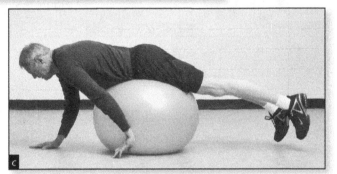

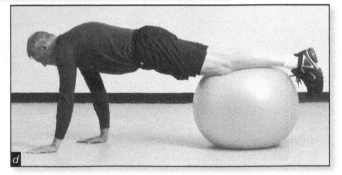

Exercise Benefits

This exercise helps to strengthen arms and shoulders before progressing to more difficult push-ups.

Hints for Various Age Levels

Only walk out as far as strength allows.

Knee Push-Up

Instructions

1. Starting position: Lie prone on the ball, with knees at the top middle of the ball.

2. Lift feet off floor and hold in a straight line with shoulders.

3. Bend arms and lower nose to the ground (see figure 9.5). Be sure to engage all muscles: Do not be a limp noodle.

4. *Note:* This version is fairly rigorous. More weight is being taken by the arms, and the body must also balance on the ball.

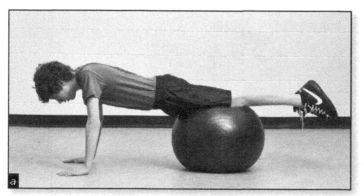

Figure 9.5   Knee Push-Up.

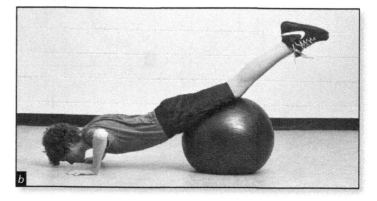

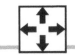

Shin Push-Up

Instructions

1. Starting position: Lie prone on the ball. Walk hands forward until shins are on the ball.
2. Lower and raise body by bending arms (see figure 9.6).

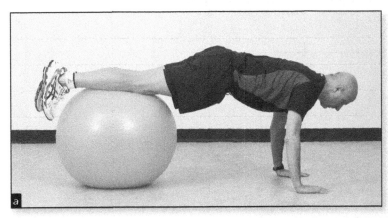

Figure 9.6 Shin Push-Up.

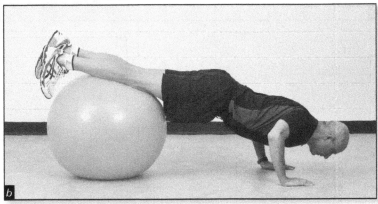

Ankle Push-Up

Instructions

1. Starting position: Lie prone on the ball. Walk hands forward until only the ankles and feet remain on the ball.

2. Execute a push-up by bending arms and lowering the body toward the floor (see figure 9.7).

3. *Note:* This push-up is for very trained and strong athletes.

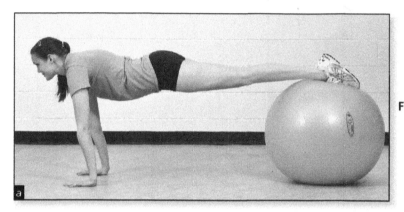

Figure 9.7 Ankle Push-Up.

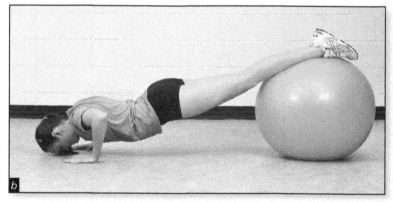

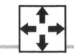

Toe Push-Up

Instructions

1. Starting position: Lie prone on the ball. Walk out until ball touches feet. Balance with toes on the ball (see figure 9.8).

2. Execute a push-up by bending arms and lowering the body toward the floor.

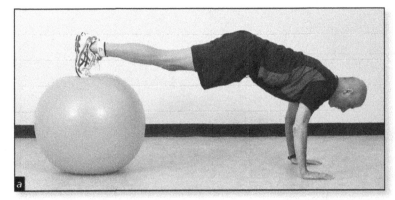

Figure 9.8 Toe Push-Up.

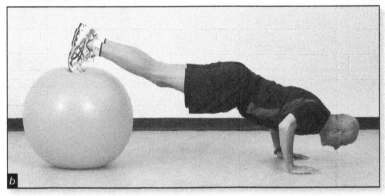

One-Leg Push-Up

Instructions

1. Starting position: Lie prone on the ball. Walk out until ball touches feet. Balance with toes on the ball. Lift one leg off the ball.

2. Execute a push-up by bending arms and lowering the body toward the floor (see figure 9.9).

3. *Note:* This is an extremely difficult exercise and needs to be worked up to.

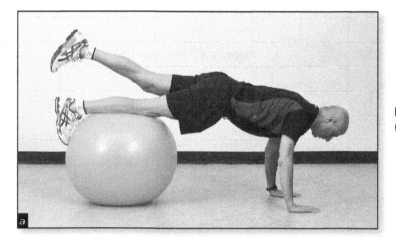

Figure 9.9   One-Leg Push-Up:
(a) start position; *(b)* lowering.

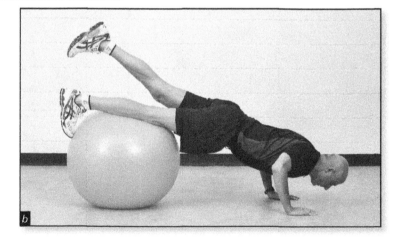

Plank

Instructions

1. Starting position: Stand directly behind the ball, with hands on ball.
2. Keep arms straight and shoulders over hands.
3. Walk feet back until the body is in the push-up position and there is a straight line from shoulders to feet (i.e., straight as a plank; see figure 9.10).
4. Hold this static position for as long as possible.

Variations

To increase the difficulty, have a partner lightly slap the ball to challenge strength and balance.

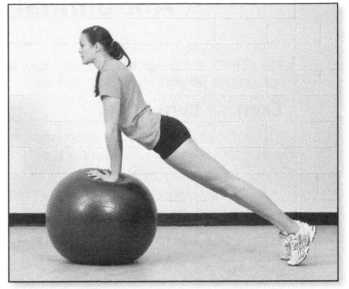

Figure 9.10   Plank.

Plank Push-Up

Instructions

1. Starting position: Stand directly behind the ball, with hands on ball.
2. Keep arms straight and shoulders over hands. Walk feet backward until in plank position.
3. Bend arms and lower the body. Stop when the arms are positioned in a right angle (see figure 9.11).
4. Return to starting position by pushing arms to the extended position.

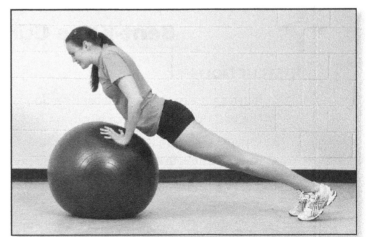

Figure 9.11   Plank Push-Up.

Muscle Group 2: Abdominal Exercises

These are some of the almost innumerable exercises for the abdominals. We tried to place them in a progression from easy to difficult, although their difficulty can be subject to a person's abilities or preference.

Exercise Benefits

The abdominal exercises strengthen the front of the torso. Core strength helps support internal organs and assists in keeping the body in an upright posture. Strong abdominal muscles are also important for back health. The muscles of the back work to support the spine and head. Together the abdominal muscles and the muscles of the back form the pelvic girdle.

Hints for Various Age Levels

Start with the first and easiest exercise and progress as your students or clients improve.

Assessment

The assessment forms for these exercises appear as full-size forms for easy printing on the bound-in CD-ROM at the back of this book.

Bent-Knee Curl/Roll-Up

Instructions

1. Starting position: Lie with back on floor, knees bent, and feet flat on floor. Hold the ball on lap and place hands on ball in front of face (see figure 9.12a).
2. Engage abdominal muscles, lift head from floor, and roll or push ball to top of knees while curling vertebrae off the floor.
3. The tips of the scapulae should lift just slightly (see figure 9.12b).

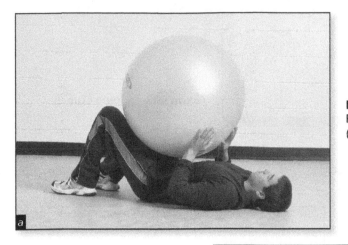

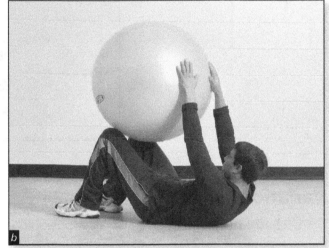

Figure 9.12 Bent-Knee Curl/Roll-Up: *(a)* starting position; *(b)* roll-up.

Supine Crunch

Instructions

1. Starting position: Lie with back on floor, calves resting on ball (see figure 9.13).
2. Lift head from floor, and curl spine upward until scapulae just leave the floor.

(continued)

Supine Crunch *(continued)*

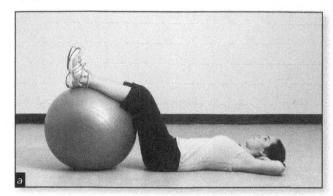

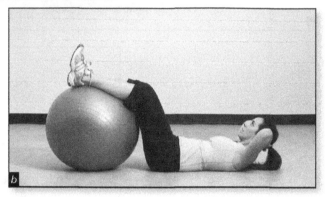

Figure 9.13 Supine Crunch.

Variations (Arms)

1. Hold arms straight forward. This position assists in transferring the weight forward.

2. Keep one arm straight in front, and support the head with the other hand (see figure 9.14). Do not pull the head with this arm. Many people find this position relaxes the neck.

3. Both hands can cradle the head and support the neck. Place hands on the back of the head. Do not lace fingers or tug on the head and neck.

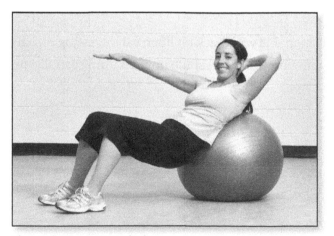

Figure 9.14 Arm variation.

Seated Mini Curl-Up

Instructions

1. Starting position: Sit on the ball. Roll the ball forward so it is at the lower back and the buttocks are slightly off the ball (see figure 9.15a).

2. Curl head and spine forward, just until scapulae leave the ball (see figure 9.15b). Arms can be held straight in front, one hand can support the head, or two hands can support the head.

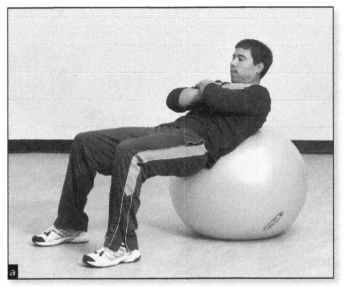

Figure 9.15 Seated Mini Curl-Up: *(a)* starting position; *(b)* ending position.

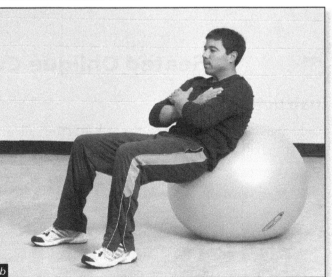

Seated Curl

Instructions

1. Starting position: Sit on the ball. Roll the ball forward so that the back is against the ball at about the two o'clock position.

2. Lean back, stretching abdominals slightly (see figure 9.16a), and then curl up.

3. Slowly roll down to start position. The muscle is then worked in both the concentric and eccentric contractions (see figure 9.16b).

4. Arms can be held straight in front, one hand can support the head, or two hands can support the head.

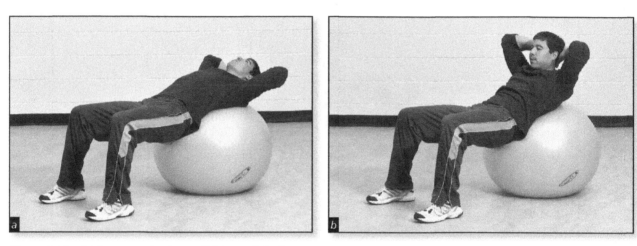

Figure 9.16 *(a)* Pre-stretch phase; *(b)* Seated Curl.

Seated Oblique Curl-Up

Instructions

1. Starting position: Sit on the ball. Roll the ball forward so that the back is against the ball at about the two o'clock position.

2. Lean back, stretching abdominals slightly.

3. Begin curl-up while reaching with one arm (or elbow) toward the opposite knee, giving a twist to the body that will work the oblique muscles (see figure 9.17).

4. Arms can be held straight in front, one hand can support the head, or two hands can support the head.

5. *Note:* Sides can be alternated for one total set, or a set can be completed on one side before doing a set on the other side.

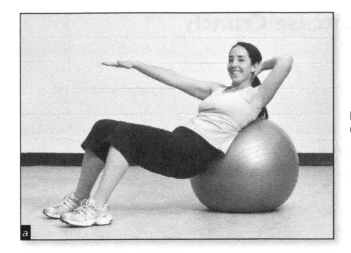

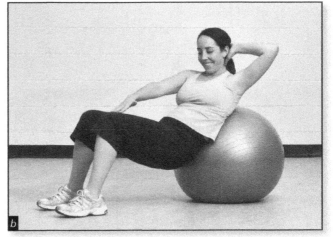

Figure 9.17 Seated Oblique Curl-Up.

Variations

Arm variations are the same as for Supine Crunch.

Suitcase Crunch

Instructions

1. Starting position: Lie on back on floor, ball under legs and tucked close to buttocks.
2. Squeeze ball with legs, and lift slightly up while curling head and spine toward knees. Scapulae should lift slightly off floor (see figure 9.18).
3. Arms can be held straight in front, one hand can support the head, or two hands can support the head.

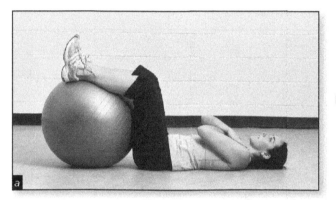

Figure 9.18   Suitcase Crunch.

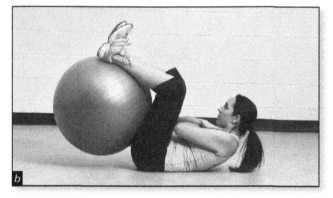

Variations

Arm variations are the same as for Supine Crunch.

Roll-Up

Instructions

1. Starting position: Lie prone on the ball in the walk-out position (see figure 9.19a).
2. Contract abdominals, and shift weight to arms.
3. Draw knees toward chest by rolling the ball with the shins and feet (see figure 9.19b).
4. Reverse the ball, and return to the extended walk-out position.
5. *Note:* This is a strenuous exercise, and the arm muscles must be strong enough to support much of the body weight. Everyone should practice Walk-Out before attempting Roll-Up.

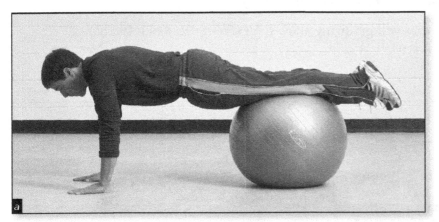

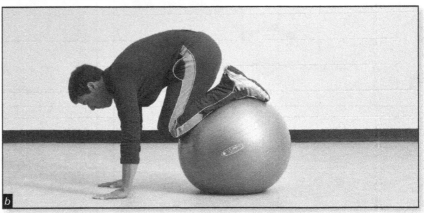

Figure 9.19 *(a)* Roll-Up starting position; *(b)* Roll-Up.

Rainbow Legs

Instructions

1. Starting position: Lie supine on the floor, with legs perpendicular to the floor. Hold the ball between the feet (see figure 9.20*a*).

2. Keeping the ball in line with the hips (do not lower legs away from head), lower the ball sideways like the arms of a metronome. Then bring legs to vertical, and lower to the other side (see figure 9.20, *b-d*).

3. *Note:* Initially two modifications should be practiced.

   • *First, bend the knees until lower legs are parallel with the floor. This shortens the metronome lever and makes it possible to perform Rainbow Legs and build the oblique abdominals.*

   • *Second, start with small movements, moving the legs from vertical just slightly until the obliques "tell" you they have had enough.*

This is a progression that will gradually allow the exerciser to touch the ball to the floor and return it to vertical.

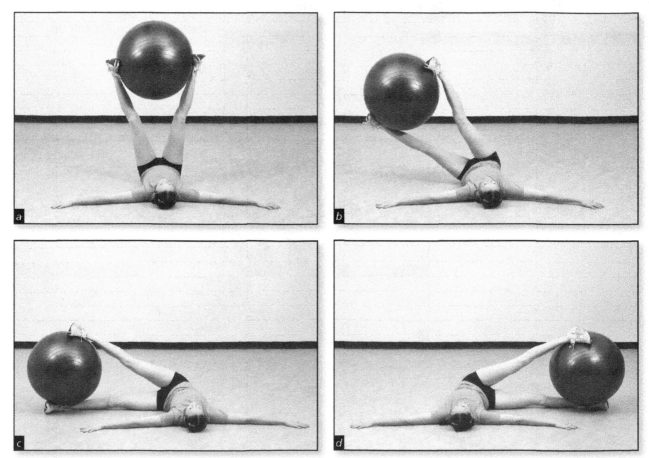

Figure 9.20 Rainbow Legs: *(a)* starting position; *(b and c)* side to side; *(d)* lower to other side.

Side-Lying Crunch

Instructions

1. Starting position: On side with knee near ball and top leg outstretched (see figure 9.21a).

2. Reach with top arm toward top foot while maintaining balance by holding ball with other hand. Side near ball lifts as opposite side does work (see figure 9.21b).

3. Do one set, and then work the other side.

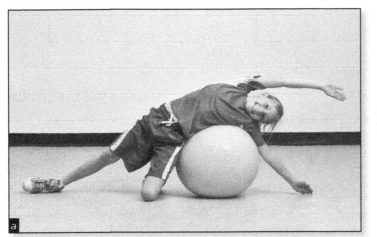

Figure 9.21 *(a)* Side-Lying Crunch starting position; *(b)* Side-Lying Crunch.

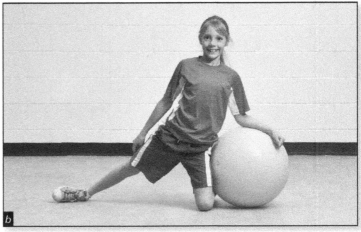

(continued)

Variations

1. Arm variation: Support head with bottom arm if balance is steady.
2. Advanced variation
   a. Starting position: On side with both legs extended. Feet can be stacked or bottom leg can be bent for better balance (see figure 9.22).
   b. Reach with top arm toward feet, raising upper torso off ball.
   c. Repeat on other side.
   d. See arm variation of Supine Crunch.

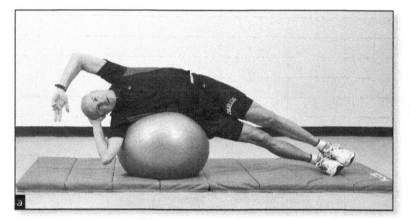

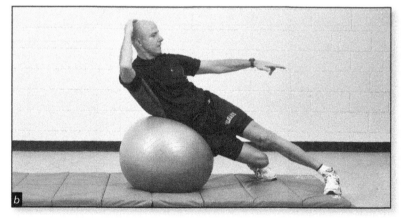

Figure 9.22   Advanced Side-Lying Crunch.

Side-Lying Crunch With Twist

Instructions

1. Starting position: On side with knee near ball and top leg outstretched (see figure 9.21a on page 129).

2. Reach toward foot while raising torso, and then twist 45 degrees to the rear (see figure 9.23a).

3. Do the same number of repetitions on other side.

Variations

1. Starting position: On side with both legs extended. Feet can be stacked or bottom leg can be bent for better balance (see figure 9.22).

2. Reach with top arm toward feet, raising upper torso off ball (see figure 9.23b).

3. Repeat on other side.

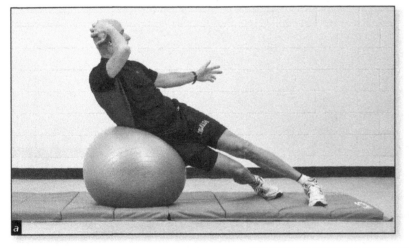

Figure 9.23 *(a)* Side-Lying Crunch With Twist; *(b)* Oblique Side-Lying Crunch.

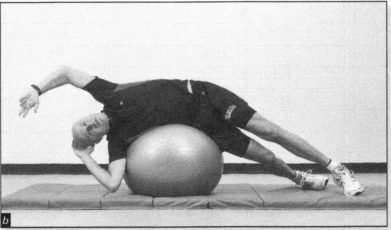

Supine Toes to Ball

Instructions

1. Starting position: Lie on back on floor, legs bent and then perpendicular to floor and ball held with extended arms above shoulders (see figure 9.24, *a* and *b*).

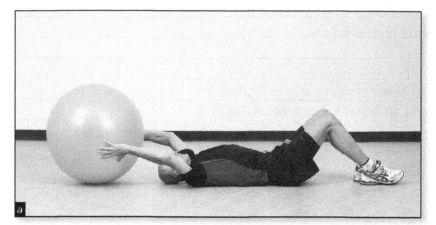

Figure 9.24 Supine Toes to Ball starting position: *(a)* legs bent; *(b)* legs perpendicular.

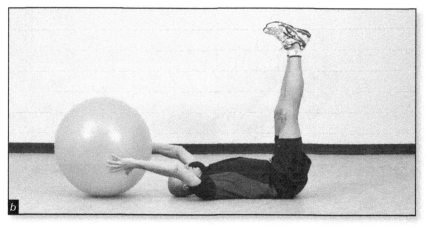

2. Bring legs toward ball using abdominals while lifting ball from the floor and holding it above the chest and belly (see figure 9.25*a*).

3. Return to start.

4. Legs may move slightly out of perpendicular toward the floor; however, caution is important to protect the back (see figure 9.25*b*).

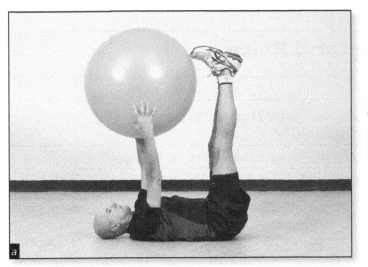

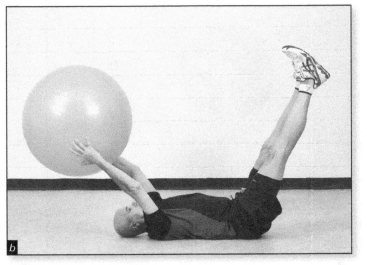

Figure 9.25 Supine Toes to Ball: *(a)* bringing legs toward ball; *(b)* legs may be slightly out of perpendicular to the floor.

Variation: One Leg

1. Starting position: Lie on back on floor, legs perpendicular to floor and ball held with extended arms above shoulders.

2. Bring one leg toward ball using abdominals while lifting ball from the floor and holding above the chest and stomach (see figure 9.26).

3. Return leg to start while moving other leg toward the ball.

4. Continue to scissor feet for 5 to 10 reps.

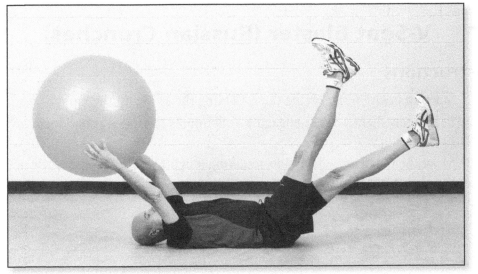

Figure 9.26 One-leg variation.

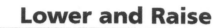

Lower and Raise

Instructions

1. Starting position: Lie on back on floor, ball held between feet with legs extended perpendicular to the floor (see figure 9.27a).
2. Bending at the knees, lower feet to a 90-degree angle (see figure 9.27b).
3. Slowly raise ball back to perpendicular.
4. Be sure to engage abdominal muscles for stability.

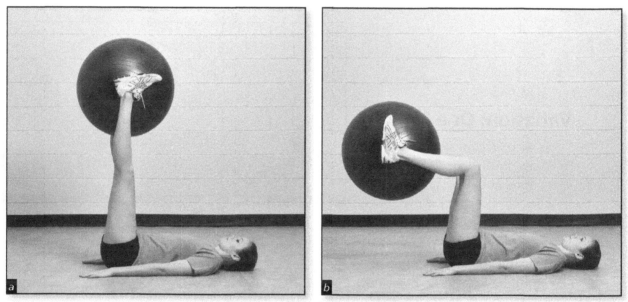

Figure 9.27 *(a)* Lower and Raise starting position; *(b)* Lower and Raise.

V-Seat Blaster (Russian Crunches)

Instructions

1. Starting position: Sit on the floor, holding the ball with the hands.
2. Lean back slightly while engaging abdominals to raise legs and form a V (see figure 9.28a).
3. Move the ball from side to side, touching it lightly to the ground while holding the V-seat position (see figure 9.28, *b* and *c*).

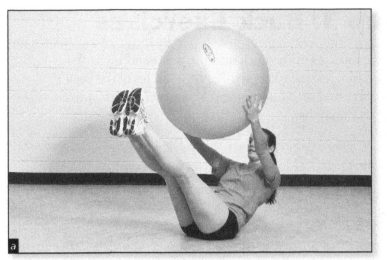

Figure 9.28 V-Seat Blaster: *(a)* starting position; *(b* and *c)* side to side.

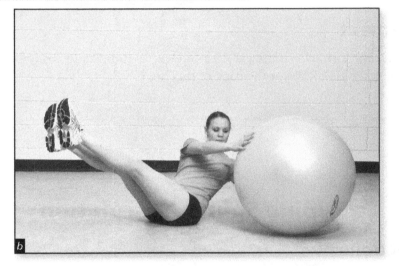

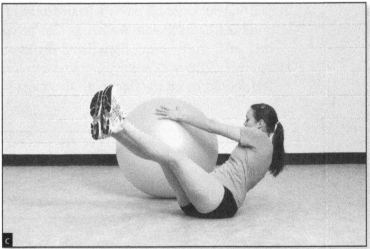

Muscle Group 3: Back Exercises

The following exercises benefit the muscles of the back and the torso and hips. The exercises are listed in a progression from easiest to most difficult. Muscles of the back include the trapezius, latissimus dorsi, and serratus anterior. The muscles of the hips are the gluteus medius, and gluteus maximus.

Exercise Benefits

The following exercises strengthen the muscles of the back and hips, and they will help prevent back problems and provide the strength for upright posture.

Hints for Various Age Levels

Take your time as you move through the progression. Do not overdo, as this can cause injury.

Assessment

 The assessment forms for these exercises appear as full-size forms for easy printing on the bound-in CD-ROM at the back of this book.

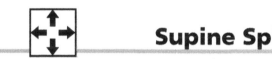

Supine Spinal Articulation

Instructions

1. Starting position: Lie on back in an extended position, arms extended overhead and holding the ball in the hands. The pelvis should be tipped so there is very little arch in the lower back. Bend the knees until this feels comfortable (see figure 9.29). *Note:* For novice or unfit persons or persons with back issues, the feet should be on the floor with the knees bent.

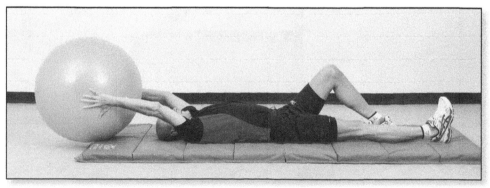

Figure 9.29 Supine Spinal Articulation starting position.

2. Raise the ball from the floor to over the head (see figure 9.30a).

3. Lift the head and spine one vertebra at a time while reaching forward with the ball (see figure 9.30b and c).

4. Reverse the action of the body and gradually, one vertebra at a time, roll back down (see figure 9.30d).

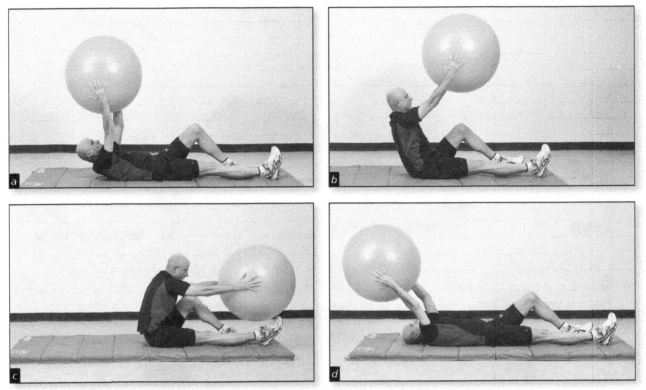

Figure 9.30 Supine Spinal Articulation: (a-c) using the ball to assist in the roll up; (d) end position.

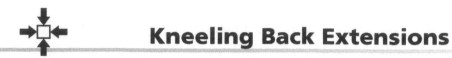

Kneeling Back Extensions

Instructions

1. Starting position: Lie prone on the ball, knees on floor (see figure 9.31a).
2. Contract abdominals and raise head and back off the ball. Do not go into an arched position.
3. At the upright position, the back will form a line between hips and shoulders (see figure 9.31b). Hold briefly and lower with control to start position.

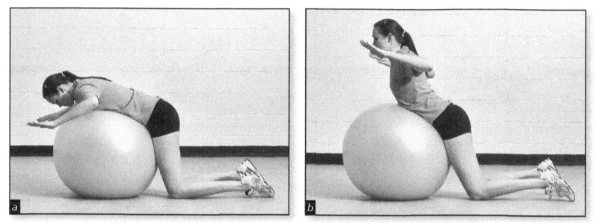

Figure 9.31 Kneeling Back Extensions: *(a)* starting position; *(b)* upright position.

Extended-Leg Back Extensions

Note: This exercise is for a person who is very experienced with Kneeling Back Extensions.

Instructions

1. Starting position: Lie prone on the ball, legs extended, feet supporting the body with the toes curled under (see figure 9.32a).
2. Raise head and back off the ball (see figure 9.32b). Do not arch the back. Hold, then return to start position.

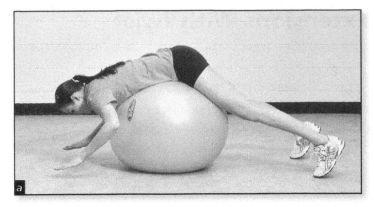

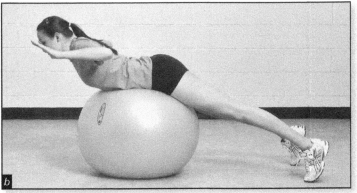

Figure 9.32 Extended-Leg Back Extensions: *(a)* starting position; *(b)* head and back off the ball.

Variations

These are arm variations for both the beginner and the experienced exerciser.

1. Arms may be held extended to the sides to form a T.
2. Arms may be held extended forward at shoulder level.
3. Arms may be held in goalpost position, bent at the elbows.

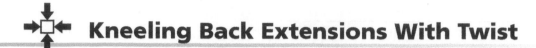

Kneeling Back Extensions With Twist

Instructions

1. Starting position: Lie prone on the ball, knees on floor (see figure 9.33a).
2. While raising the head and back, twist spine and look to side (see figure 9.33b).
3. Keep hips on the ball, and twist only as far as comfortable.
4. Lower to starting position.
5. Repeat on other side.

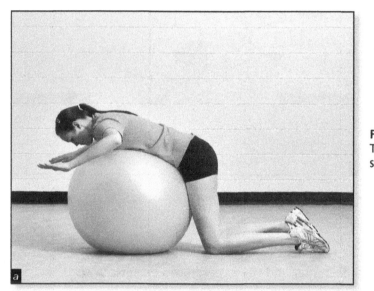

Figure 9.33 Kneeling Back Extensions With Twist: *(a)* starting position; *(b)* twisting to the side.

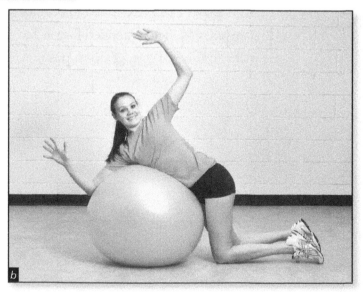

Extended-Leg Back Extensions With Twist

Note: This exercise is for a person who is very experienced with Kneeling Back Extensions With Twist.

Instructions

1. Starting position: Lie prone on the ball, legs extended, feet supporting the body with the toes curled under (see figure 9.32*a* on page 139).

2. Raise head and back off the ball (see figure 9.32*b* on page 139). Do not arch the back. Hold, then return to start position.

3. While raising head and back, twist spine and look to side (see figure 9.34).

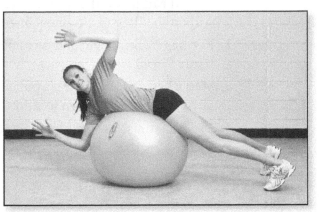

Figure 9.34 Extended-Leg Back Extensions With Twist.

4. Keep hips on the ball; do not roll to the side.

5. The options for arm position can be straight ahead, out to the side in a T, or bent at the elbows to form a goalpost.

Grasshopper

Instructions

1. Starting position: Kneel behind the ball about 12 to 15 inches (30 to 38 cm) away. Lean forward and rest forearms on the ball with feet in the air, knees still on the floor (see figure 9.35a).

2. Keeping back straight and pressing hips forward, slowly roll the ball away (see figure 9.35b).

3. Stop when you start to feel a pull in your back muscles. Do not roll too far. You need to be able to return to start.

4. Use back muscles to return to start.

5. This exercise also uses abdominal muscles. Be sure to hold all muscles tight.

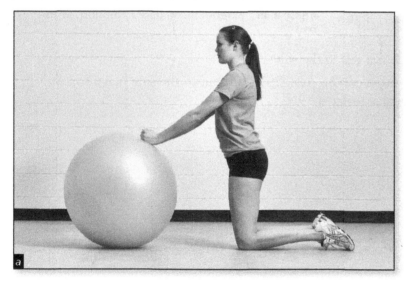

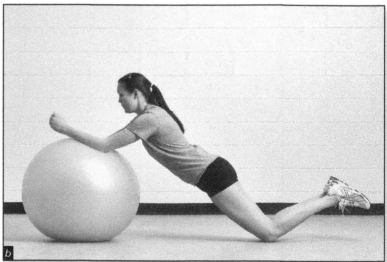

Figure 9.35 Grasshopper: *(a)* starting position; *(b)* slowly rolling the ball away.

Muscle Group 4: Hamstring Exercises

The **hamstrings** are located on the back of the thigh (upper leg). Consisting of the biceps femoris, semimembranosus, and semitendinosus, they act opposite to the quadriceps. The exercises in this section focus on strengthening the hamstrings.

Exercise Benefits

The following exercises strengthen the hamstrings.

Assessment

The assessment forms for these exercises appear as full-size forms for easy printing on the bound-in CD-ROM at the back of this book.

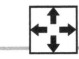

Supine Roll-Outs

Instructions

1. Starting position: Lie on back on the floor, knees bent and feet on the ball (see figure 9.36*a*).

2. Keeping head and back on the floor, roll the ball away from the body with the feet. Then roll it back to the starting position (see figure 9.36*b*).

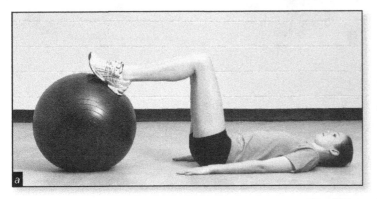

Figure 9.36 Supine Roll-Out: *(a)* starting position; *(b)* rolling the ball away from the body with the feet.

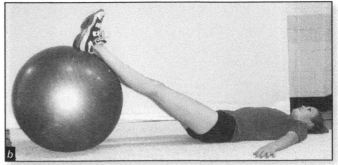

© Anne Spalding

Hip Lift

Instructions

1. Starting position: Lie on back on the floor, knees bent and feet on the ball (see figure 9.37a).

2. Contract abdominal muscles and press feet into the ball, lifting back until the body forms a straight line with the shoulders (see figure 9.37b).

3. Lower slowly to the floor.

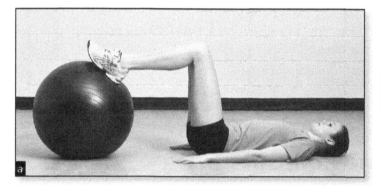

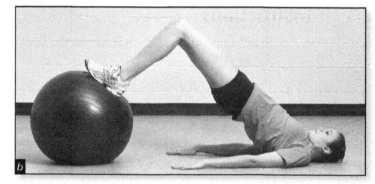

Figure 9.37 Hip Lift: *(a)* starting position; *(b)* lifting back until the body forms a straight line.

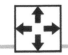

Hamstring Combination

Instructions

1. Starting position: Lie on back on the floor, knees bent and feet on the ball (see figure 9.36a on page 143).

2. Lift hips as in Hip Lift. Keeping hips lifted, roll the ball away (see figure 9.38a).

3. Next pull the ball back to the hip-lift position, and then lower the hips slowly (see figure 9.38b).

4. *Note:* This is a very strenuous exercise, and both Supine Roll-Outs and Hip Lift should be mastered before attempting Hamstring Combination.

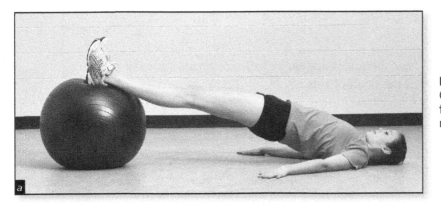

Figure 9.38 Hamstring Combination: *(a)* lying on back, feet on the ball; *(b)* hamstring roll-out.

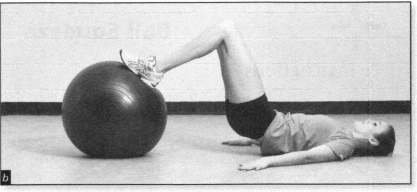

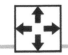

Hummers

Instructions

1. Starting position: Lie on back on the floor, knees bent and feet on the ball (see figure 9.36a on page 143).

2. Begin with Hip Lift, then do a roll-out.

3. Do not lower the hips after returning to the hip-lift position, but continue to roll the ball out and in (see figure 9.38b on this page).

4. *Note:* This exercise is aptly named because your hamstrings will be humming when you finish.

Muscle Group 5:
Inner Thighs Exercises

The muscles of the inner thighs are referred to as adductors because they bring the legs together. The adductors consist of the pectineus, adductor brevis, adductor longus, and adductor magnus.

Exercise Benefits

The following exercises strengthen the adductors.

Hints for Various Age Levels

Enjoy these fun exercises.

Assessment

The assessment forms for these exercises appear as full-size forms for easy printing on the bound-in CD-ROM at the back of this book.

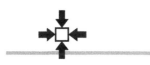

Ball Squeeze

Instructions

1. Starting position: Lie on back on the floor, legs raised perpendicular to the floor and holding the ball between the feet (see figure 9.39).

2. Using the adductors (inner thighs), squeeze the ball as tightly as possible, hold for two seconds, and relax but don't let the ball fall.

3. Repeat.

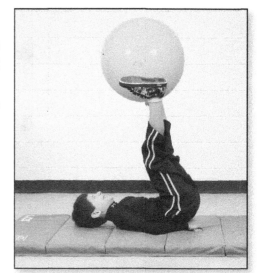

Figure 9.39 Ball Squeeze.

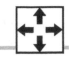

Ball Toss and Catch

Instructions

1. Starting position: Lie on back on the floor, legs raised perpendicular to the floor and holding the ball between the feet.
2. Release the ball with the feet and hold in hands.
3. Toss the ball one to two feet (30 to 61 cm) above the feet and in such a trajectory that it will fall straight down to feet (see figure 9.40).
4. Catch the ball with the feet, and squeeze the ball as in Ball Squeeze.
5. Release the ball to the hands and repeat.

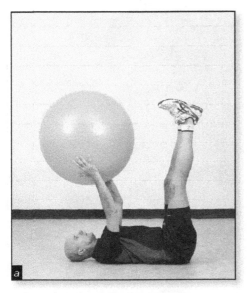
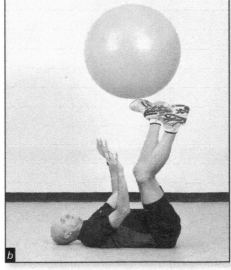

Figure 9.40 Ball Toss and Catch.

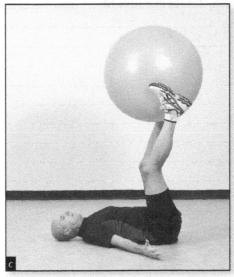

Instructions

1. Starting position: Lie on back on the floor, legs raised perpendicular to the floor, holding the ball between the feet. Place arms on floor with hands slightly away from the sides, forming a V (see figure 9.41*a*).

2. With feet rotate the ball until feet are at 12 and 6 o'clock (see figure 9.41*b*).

3. Then twist (rotate) the ball until the feet are reversed (see figure 9.41*c*).

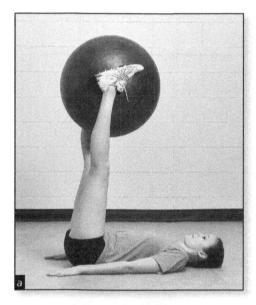
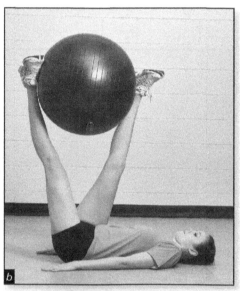
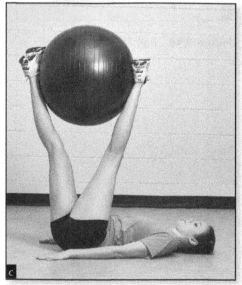

Figure 9.41 Twisties: *(a)* starting position; *(b)* with feet at 12 and 6; *(c)* with feet at 6 and 12.

Muscle Group 6:
Leg Combinations—Quadriceps, Hamstrings, Inner Thighs Exercises

The exercises described in this section involve all muscles of the upper leg: **quadriceps** (front of thigh), hamstrings (rear of thigh), and inner thigh. While these exercises look easy, be sure to perform them mindfully. Froggie and Prone Bend and Lift are subtle and difficult to do.

Exercise Benefits

These exercises strengthen the muscles of the upper leg: hamstrings, inner thighs, and quadriceps.

Variations

The Rear Lunge and Side Lunge have variations; otherwise, there are no variations for the other exercises.

Hints for Various Age Levels

Start with small movements and be aware of the subtle lift for Froggie and Prone Bend and Lift. The two lunge exercises should be done to the best of the performer's ability and gradually improved.

Assessment

The assessment forms for these exercises appear as full-size forms for easy printing on the bound-in CD-ROM at the back of this book.

Froggie

Instructions

1. Starting position: Lie prone on the ball, hands on the floor and soles of feet touching in the air, with knees slightly bent (see figure 9.42*a*).

2. Raise feet toward ceiling (see figure 9.42*b*), and then lower slowly toward the floor. Do not touch the floor with the feet.

3. Repeat.

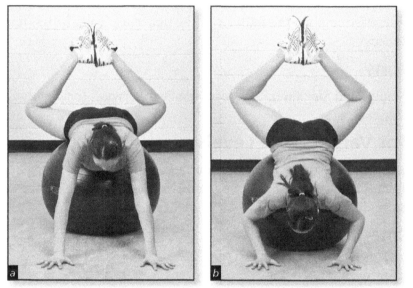

Figure 9.42 Froggie: *(a)* starting position; *(b)* raising feet toward ceiling.

Prone Bend and Lift

Instructions

1. Starting position: Lie prone on the ball in the walk-out position (hands on floor, feet off floor, hips on ball, and knees bent; see figure 9.43a).
2. Contract quadriceps, and lift feet toward ceiling (see figure 9.43b).
3. Hold, then lower legs and repeat.
4. *Note:* Only a slight lift occurs.

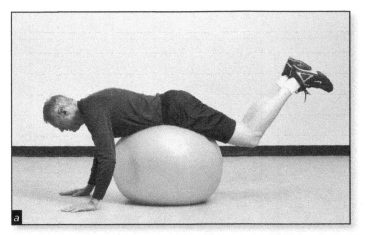

Figure 9.43 Prone Bend and Lift: *(a)* starting position; *(b)* lifting feet toward ceiling.

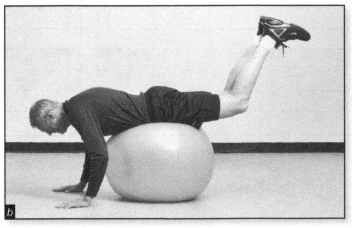

Rear Lunge

Instructions

1. Starting position: Stand on one leg with the ball to the side. The middle of the ball is in line with the heel of the supporting leg. Rest the shin on the ball (see figure 9.44a).

2. Bend the knee of the standing (supporting) leg while rolling the ball to the rear with the shin of the other leg. The upper body should lean forward but remain upright (see figure 9.44b).

3. Return to starting position and repeat. Be sure to work the other leg.

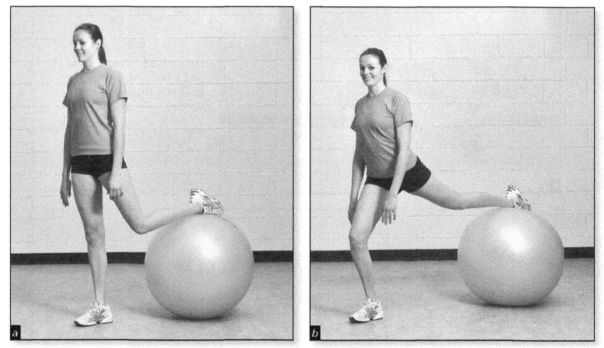

Figure 9.44 Rear Lunge: *(a)* starting position; *(b)* rolling ball to rear with shin.

Variation: Advanced Rear Lunge

This exercise is for someone who is very experienced with the original Rear Lunge exercise.

1. Starting position: Stand on one leg as in Rear Lunge. Place the nonsupporting foot on the top of the ball (see figure 9.45a).

2. Bend the knee of the supporting leg while rolling the ball backward until the leg is fully extended (see figure 9.45b).

3. Return to starting position by rolling the ball forward with the foot.

4. Repeat exercise, and then switch to the other leg.

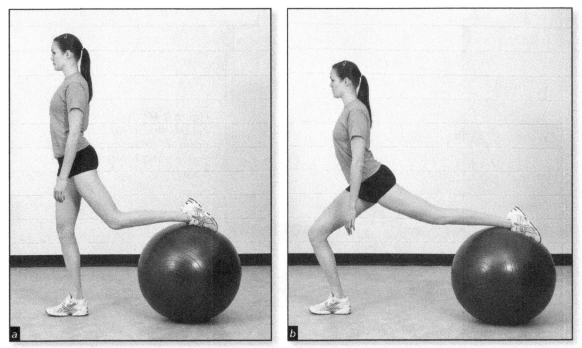

Figure 9.45 Advanced Rear Lunge: *(a)* starting position; *(b)* leg is fully extended.

Rear Lunge Pebble Pickup

Instructions

1. Starting position: Stand on one leg as in Rear Lunge. Place the nonsupporting foot on top of the ball (see figure 9.46a).
2. Bend the knee of the supporting leg while rolling the ball backward until the leg is fully extended.
3. While in the lunge position for either beginner or experienced, lean forward toward floor and pick up an imaginary pebble (see figure 9.46b).
4. Return upper body to upright position, and return to start.

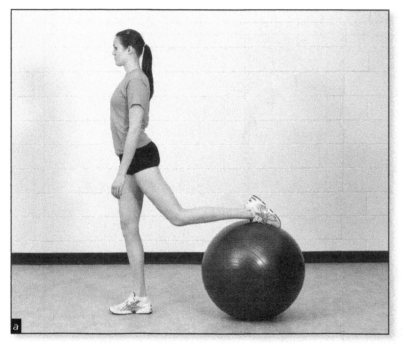

Figure 9.46 Rear Lunge Pebble Pickup: *(a)* starting position; *(b)* lunge position and leaning forward toward floor.

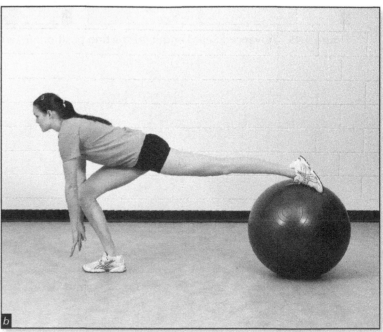

Instructions

1. Starting position: Stand on one leg with the ball to the other side. Place foot of nonsupporting leg on top of the ball (see figure 9.47a).

2. Bend knee of supporting leg while rolling the ball sideways until the leg is extended fully (see figure 9.47b).

3. Keep upper body upright as much as possible.

4. Slowly roll ball to the starting position. Repeat, then work other leg.

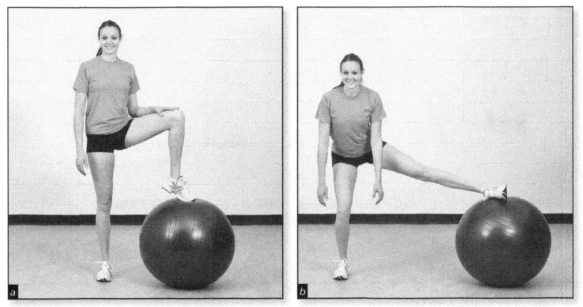

Figure 9.47 Side Lunge: *(a)* starting position; *(b)* rolling ball sideways until leg is fully extended.

(continued)

Variation: Foot Touch With Side Lunge

1. Starting position: Stand on one leg with the ball to the other side. Place foot of nonsupporting leg on top of the ball (see figure 9.48*a*).

2. Bend knee of supporting leg while rolling the ball sideways until the leg is extended fully (see figure 9.48*b*).

3. In the lunge position, bend upper body to the side, and try to touch the side of the foot (see figure 9.48*c*).

4. Return to upright position, and return to the starting position.

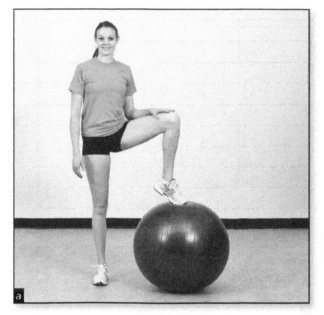
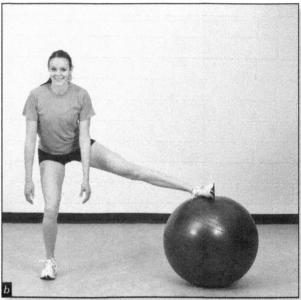

Figure 9.48 Foot Touch With Side Lunge: *(a)* starting position; *(b)* rolling ball sideways until leg is extended fully; *(c)* trying to touch side of foot.

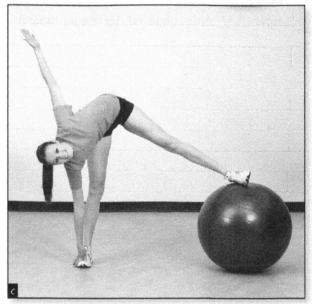

Flexibility Exercises

• •

Flexibility is the range of motion (ROM) through which each joint is capable of moving. It is critical for all motor skills and is part of the foundation of athletic excellence. Everyone needs a minimum level of flexibility for efficient and effective daily functioning, and the exercise ball is an excellent piece of equipment to use for increasing flexibility. An exercise ball is supportive and elastic at the same time, and it allows exercisers to be supported and comfortable while stretching. Often stretching can be viewed as tedious; however, with the exercise ball, it becomes fun and challenging play rather than work.

To maintain flexibility, you should stretch a minimum of three times a week. If you use the exercise ball for a stand-alone flexibility workout, be sure to do a general body warm-up—such as walking for 5 to 10 minutes or jogging for 5 minutes or bouncing on the exercise ball—to get muscles prepared and warmed up for stretching.

Following are some guidelines for stretching:

1. Stretch slowly, and *do not* bounce.
2. Stop the stretch when you feel tension in the muscle you are stretching (the point of tightness).
3. Hold the stretch for 15 seconds or longer.
4. Exhale during the hold, and attempt to relax the muscle.
5. Repeat the stretch two to five times.
6. *Do not* stretch to the point of pain.
7. Everyone's flexibility is different.
8. Stretching is not a competition. This is one example of how injuries can occur.
9. Additional stretching repetitions will improve flexibility, as will daily stretching.

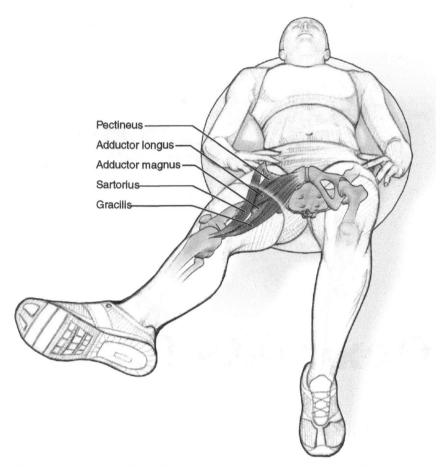

Pectineus

Adductor longus

Adductor magnus

Sartorius

Gracilis

Muscles used during flexibility exercises. Using the exercise ball helps to increase flexibility.

Another type of stretching similar to the **static stretching** outlined in the previous list is active isolated stretching, or **AIS**. Aaron Mattes (www.stretchingusa.com) developed this technique, which often works more quickly than static stretching. For simplicity, we can say it is similar to standard stretching. AIS is based on the premise that the stretch reflex—which occurs within about two seconds of reaching the tension point of the stretch—protects the stretched muscle from tearing and prevents the muscle from stretching past the point of maximal stretch. Therefore, no further stretch can occur once the stretch reflex occurs. In the AIS method, repeated stretches are done and held for only two seconds. The steps in AIS are as follows:

1. Contract the **agonist muscle** (the muscle opposite from the one you are stretching). This allows the muscle you want to stretch to relax and stretch.

2. After reaching the point of tension, gently assist the stretch (with a strap, by a partner, or by yourself).

3. Hold the stretch for two seconds by counting, "One Mississippi, two Mississippi," and then release the stretch and return the body part to the initial position.

4. Repeat this procedure for 8 to 15 repetitions.

Returning the muscle to the original position ensures that the muscle receives blood and oxygen. Completing the 8 to 15 repetitions means that the stretching takes approximately the same amount of time as static stretching. The advantage is a minute increase in muscle length with each repetition.

Each of the exercises in this chapter can be used as a stand-alone stretch. However, we usually incorporate them into an exercise ball workout immediately after the end of a strength exercise, thereby combining strength training and stretching of a muscle group. Another option is to do group stretches at the end of an exercise ball workout to stretch the muscles used during the workout.

Prone Stretch

Instructions

1. Starting position: Assume a basic prone position with the chin resting on the ball, hands on ball near the face as if in a resting position.
2. Keeping knees anchored to the floor, roll the ball forward by elongating the spine.
3. Exhale as the ball rolls forward, and relax into this stretch (see figure 10.1).
4. *Note:* This is a subtle but powerful stretch. It opens the spaces between the vertebrae that become compacted by gravity as a result of our upright posture.
5. Many exercisers will push with the feet, lifting the knees from the floor. As a result they will not feel any stretch. This is very much a mindful stretch and should be revisited until each student says, "Aha!"

Exercise Benefits

Flexibility of the spine and elongation of the spine which keeps the vertebrae from compressing.

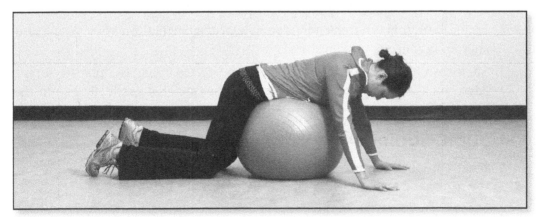

Figure 10.1   Prone Stretch.

(continued)

Hints for Various Age Levels

Rock back on heels before rolling forward. It will give more of a sense of the spinal elongation.

Assessment

The assessment form for this exercise appears as a full-size form for easy printing on the bound-in CD-ROM at the back of this book.

Supine Arch (Spinal Stretch)

Instructions

1. Starting position: Sit on the ball (see figure 10.2*a*).
2. Walk feet forward while rolling spine backward over the ball. Hands should be by the sides of the ball to provide stability if necessary (see figure 10.2*b* and *c*).
3. *Note:* For some people with very rigid spines, there will be no curvature in the spine, and this position will be very uncomfortable (see figure 10.2*d*). Work with these persons, and remind them to stop if they feel pain because they have stretched too far. For others, this inverted position is awkward and scary. These people will need to be spotted the first time or two (see figure 10.2*e*).

Exercise Benefits

1. Supine Arch expands the vertebral column much like an inversion apparatus does, but with more support. This expansion allows better blood flow to the spinal nerves and compensates for our frequent hunched-over postures that we hold when sitting at desks and especially computers.
2. In addition, this is a tremendous stretch for the pectoral muscles, which also shorten because of desk posture.
3. Supine Arch can be combined with the next stretch (which is opposite Supine Arch) by alternating the two in a series of sweeps that gradually loosen the spine.

Variation: Supine Arch With Chest Stretch

1. Make sure the head is on the ball and supported, not lifted and held flexed at the neck.
2. Spread arms away from the body, opening the chest area (see figure 10.3*a*). If comfortable, sweep the arms to an extended position over the head, as if making a snow angel (see figure 10.3*b*).

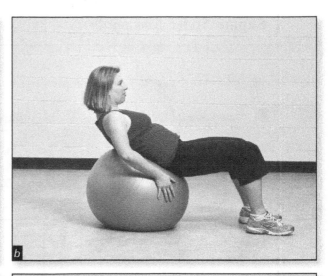

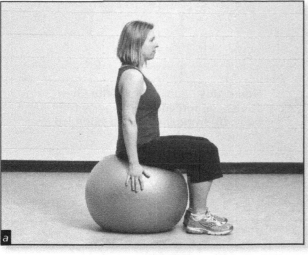

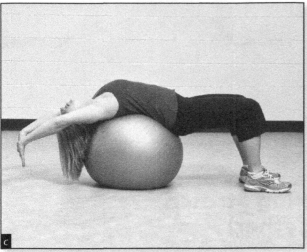

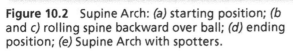

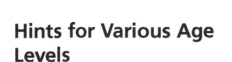

Figure 10.2 Supine Arch: *(a)* starting position; *(b and c)* rolling spine backward over ball; *(d)* ending position; *(e)* Supine Arch with spotters.

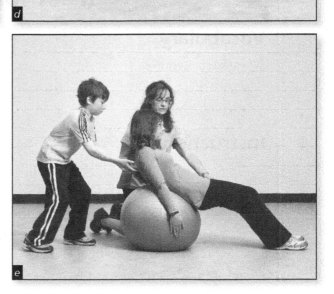

Hints for Various Age Levels

This is a powerful stretch. Check to make sure students or clients are comfortable being upside down. Some people will need spotting when doing this exercise.

Assessment

The assessment form for this exercise appears as a full-size form for easy printing on the bound-in CD-ROM at the back of this book.

(continued)

Supine Arch *(continued)*

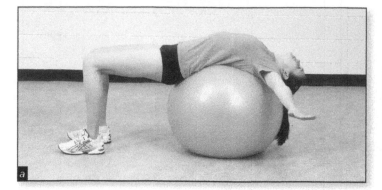

Figure 10.3 Supine Arch With Chest Stretch: *(a)* spreading arms away from body; *(b)* sweeping arms to extended position over the head.

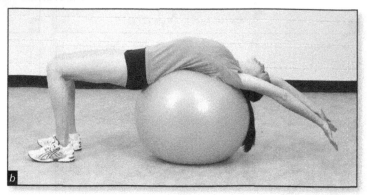

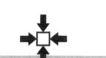

Seated Hamstring Stretch (Feet Together)

Vocabulary

- gastrocnemius
- soleus
- biceps femoris

Instructions

1. Starting position: Sit on the ball.
2. With knees bent, lean forward and grasp feet over toes or around side of feet, with fingers holding the ball of the foot (see figure 10.4*a*).
3. Keeping heels on the floor, slowly push the ball away from the feet, gradually extending legs (see figure 10.4*b*).
4. Stop when tension is felt, and exhale (see figure 10.4*c*).
5. Release feet and return to the seated position.

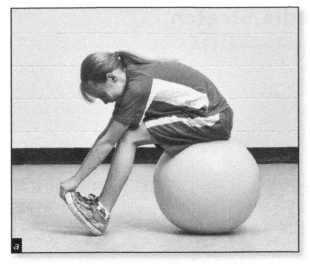

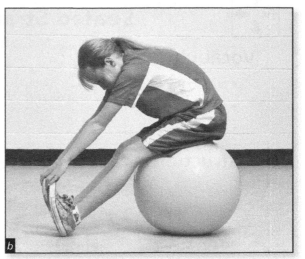

Figure 10.4 Seated Hamstring Stretch: *(a)* leaning forward to grasp feet; *(b)* pushing ball away from feet; *(c)* stopping and exhaling when tension is felt.

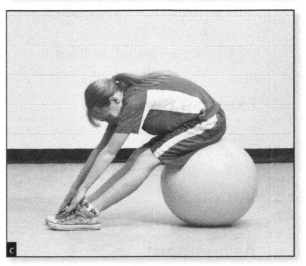

Exercise Benefits

This exercise stretches all muscles in the back of both the upper and lower legs and the low back, including the **gastrocnemius**, **soleus**, **biceps femoris**, gluteus, and erector spinae.

Variations

If combining this stretch with Supine Arch, alternate each stretch and repeat four to eight times. Also, see Seated Straddle Stretch on page 164.

Hints for Various Age Levels

Because many people have "tight" hamstrings, caution them to move slowly and to stop at the point of tension. If the stretch starts to hurt, they have stretched too far.

Assessment

The assessment form for this exercise appears as a full-size form for easy printing on the bound-in CD-ROM at the back of this book.

Seated Straddle Stretch

Vocabulary

- adductors
- gracilis
- pectineus

Instructions

1. Starting position: Sit on the ball with legs extended in a straddle position (see figure 10.5a).
2. Bending from the hips, fold body in half (as best as possible) by reaching to the floor (see figure 10.5b).
3. Stop and hold when tension is felt. Fingers might touch the floor or not (see figure 10.5c).
4. Some people will be able to touch hands flat to the floor (see figure 10.5d), and some people can put forearms on the floor (see figure 10.5e).

Exercise Benefits

This exercise enhances flexibility of the hips, back, and legs (gluteus, biceps femoris, gastrocnemius, and soleus) and the inner thigh muscles (**adductors**, longus and magnus, **gracilis**, and **pectineus**).

Variations

See Seated Hamstring Stretch on page 162.

Assessment

The assessment form for this exercise appears as a full-size form for easy printing on the bound-in CD-ROM at the back of this book.

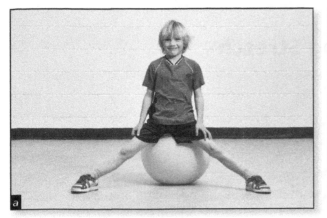
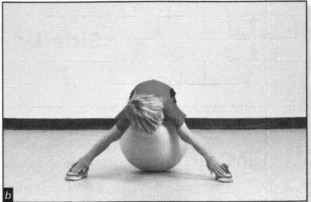
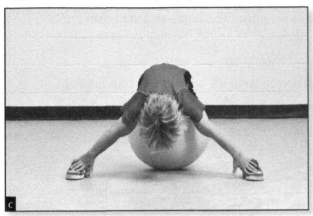
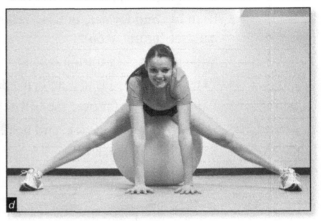
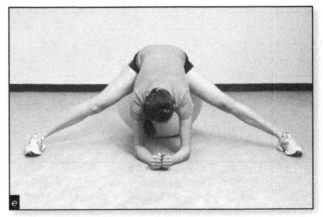

Figure 10.5 Seated Straddle Stretch: *(a)* starting position; *(b)* folding body toward floor; *(c)* holding when tension is felt; *(d)* hands flat on floor; *(e)* forearms on floor.

Side-Lying Stretch

Vocabulary

- obliquus abdominis
- serratus anterior

Instructions

1. Starting position: Kneel on the floor with the ball at the side, hand on the ball (see figure 10.6a).
2. Lean hip and lay side of torso on the ball, sliding the hand and arm over the ball (see figure 10.6b).
3. Straighten top leg until it extends straight from hip (see figure 10.6c).
4. Extend lower leg (as in Side-Lying Balance on page 85, which is a prerequisite).
5. Extend body as far over the ball as possible by pulling arms away from feet.
6. Stop when tension is felt, and hold.
7. Repeat on other side.

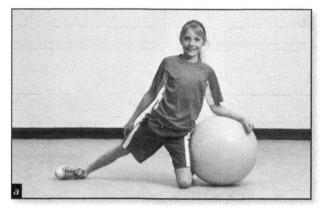
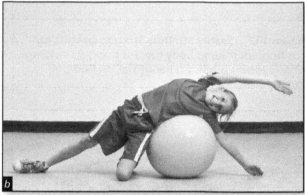
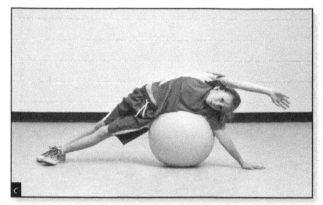

Figure 10.6 Side-Lying Stretch: *(a)* extending lower leg; *(b)* extending body as far over ball as possible; *(c)* holding when tension is felt.

Exercise Benefits

This exercise increases flexibility in abdominal obliques and transverse abdominals, and stretches the **obliquus abdominis**, **serratus anterior**, and gluteus medius.

Hints for Various Age Levels

Be sure the student or client can perform the Side-Lying Balance before attempting this stretch.

Assessment

The assessment form for this exercise appears as a full-size form for easy printing on the bound-in CD-ROM at the back of this book.

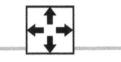 # Straddle Stand

Vocabulary

None.

Instructions

1. Starting position: Stand in a straddle position, with ball on floor in front of body and hands on ball (see figure 10.7a).
2. Bending from the waist, roll the ball away until back is parallel with floor or until tension is felt in inner thighs and lower back (see figure 10.7b).
3. To intensify the stretch, be sure head is between arms and looking downward.

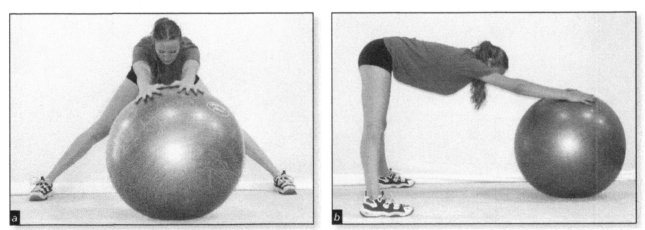

Figure 10.7 Straddle Stand: *(a)* starting position; *(b)* rolling the ball away.
© Anne Spalding

Exercise Benefits

This exercise stretches muscles of the inner thigh (adductor longus and magnus, gracilis, and pectineus), the lower back (erector spinae), and the gluteus.

Assessment

The assessment form for this exercise appears as a full-size form for easy printing on the bound-in CD-ROM at the back of this book.

Quadriceps Stretch

Instructions

1. Starting position: Lie prone on the ball, hands and feet touching floor (see figure 10.8a).
2. Bend one knee, moving foot as close to buttocks as possible (see figure 10.8b).
3. With arm on the same side, reach back and grab ankle (see figure 10.8c).
4. Slowly and gently, lift foot toward ceiling (see figure 10.8d).
5. Stop at the point of tightness and hold.
6. Release and repeat. Then stretch other leg.

Exercise Benefits

This exercise stretches the quadriceps muscles.

Hints for Various Age Levels

This can be a difficult stretch for some students or clients. Assistance may be necessary to grab the ankle.

Assessment

The assessment form for this exercise appears as a full-size form for easy printing on the bound-in CD-ROM at the back of this book.

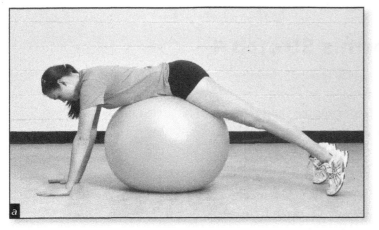

Figure 10.8 Quadriceps Stretch: *(a)* starting position; *(b)* moving foot toward buttocks; *(c)* grabbing ankle; *(d)* lifting foot toward ceiling.

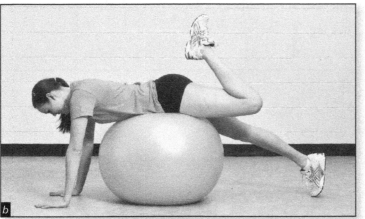

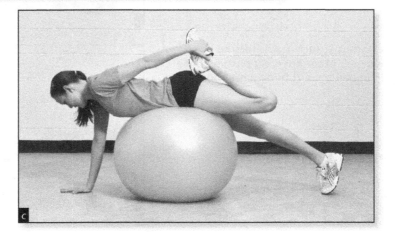

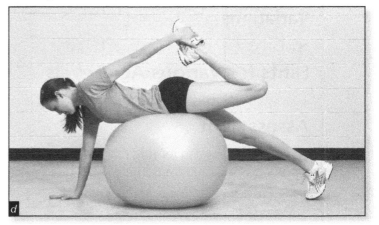

Piriformis Stretch 1

Instructions

1. Starting position: Lie on the floor supine (belly up), with both feet on ball and knees bent. The exercise ball will be about 12 to 18 inches (30 to 45 cm) from the buttocks (see figure 10.9a).

2. Cross ankle of one leg over knee of other leg (see figure 10.9b).

3. With hand nearest bent knee, gently push knee away while pulling the ball toward the body with the opposite foot (see figure 10.9c).

4. Stop when tightness is felt, and hold.

5. Repeat with other leg.

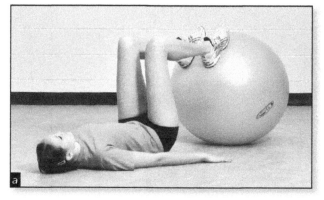
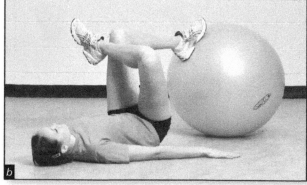

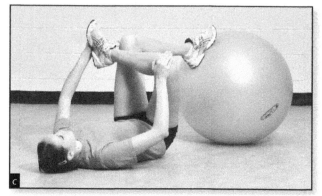

Figure 10.9 Piriformis Stretch 1: *(a)* starting position; *(b)* crossing ankle over other knee; *(c)* pushing knee away while pulling ball toward body with opposite foot.

Exercise Benefits

This exercise stretches the piriformis and other rotator muscles of the hip used in running and kicking.

Variations

See Piriformis Stretch 2 on page 171.

Hints for Various Age Levels

This stretch feels terrific. Be sure to repeat it several times.

Assessment

The assessment form for this exercise appears as a full-size form for easy printing on the bound-in CD-ROM at the back of this book.

Piriformis Stretch 2

Instructions

1. Starting position: Sit on the ball, dropping buttocks toward floor so that lower back is resting against the ball (see figure 10.10a).
2. Cross ankle of one leg over knee of other leg (see figure 10.10b).
3. Continue to roll down ball until tightness is felt (see figure 10.10c).
4. Hands can be placed on floor for balance. Stop and hold stretch.
5. Roll back to seated position.
6. Repeat with other leg.

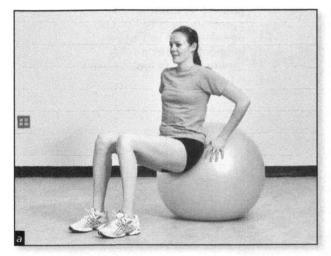 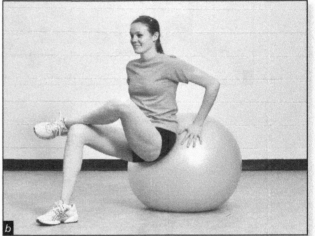

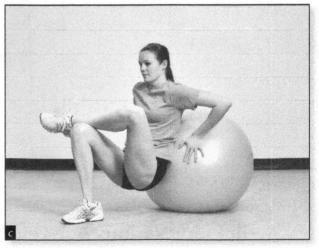

Figure 10.10 Piriformis Stretch 2: (a) starting position; (b) crossing ankle over other knee; (c) rolling down ball until tightness is felt.

Exercise Benefits

This exercise stretches the piriformis and other rotator muscles of the hip used in running and kicking.

Variations

See Piriformis Stretch 1 on page 170.

Hints for Various Age Levels

This stretch feels terrific. Be sure to repeat it several times.

Assessment

The assessment form for this exercise appears as a full-size form for easy printing on the bound-in CD-ROM at the back of this book.

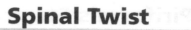

Spinal Twist

Instructions

1. Starting position: Lie on back on the floor. Place feet on the floor with knees bent. Hold ball on floor above head (see figure 10.11*a*).
2. Drop both knees to floor on one side of body while rolling ball in opposite direction (see figure 10.11*b*).
3. Turn head to look at ball (see figure 10.11*c*).

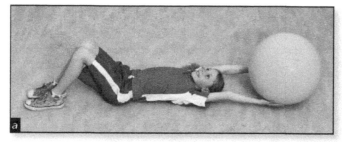

Figure 10.11 Spinal Twist: *(a)* starting position; *(b)* dropping knees to floor on one side while rolling ball in opposite direction; *(c)* turning head to look at ball.

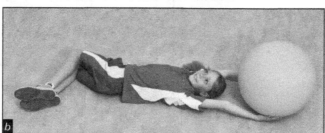

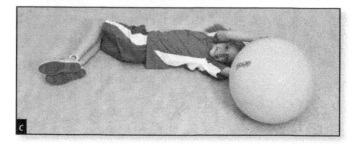

Exercise Benefits

This exercise stretches muscles of the lower back and hip.

Hints for Various Age Levels

This is a stretch that everyone can do. It also feels terrific.

Assessment

The assessment form for this exercise appears as a full-size form for easy printing on the bound-in CD-ROM at the back of this book.

Hip Flexor Stretch

Instructions

1. Starting position: Kneel with one knee on floor, with hands on the ball in front of body. Place one foot at the side of the ball, and lean forward onto ball while extending other leg (see figure 10.12*a*). The position should be like a lunge supported by the ball.

2. Tuck toe under and rock back, as if trying to touch heel to the floor and straightening leg until tension is felt in the hip flexor. To increase the stretch, roll the ball forward (see figure 10.12*b*).

3. Be sure not to let bent knee go in front of toes (past a 90-degree angle). Avoid injury to the knee by moving this foot forward.

4. Hold stretch, and then repeat with other leg.

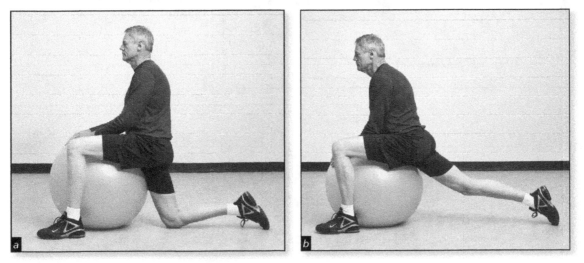

Figure 10.12 Hip Flexor Stretch: *(a)* starting position; *(b)* lunge supported by the ball.

Exercise Benefits

This exercise increases flexibility in hip flexors.

Hints for Various Age Levels

Be sure to stress keeping the foot in front of the knee.

Assessment

The assessment form for this exercise appears as a full-size form for easy printing on the bound-in CD-ROM at the back of this book.

Gastrocnemius Stretch

Instructions

1. Starting position: Lie prone on the ball, hands on floor, legs extended. Tuck toes of one foot under, and place other foot on top at heel (see figure 10.13*a*).
2. Roll the ball backward while pressing with top foot.
3. Stretch the gastrocnemius by trying to touch the sole of foot to the floor (see figure 10.13*b*).

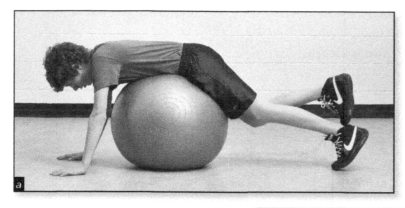

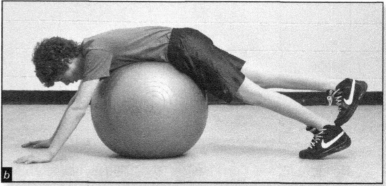

Figure 10.13 Gastrocnemius Stretch: *(a)* starting position; *(b)* pressing heel to floor.

Exercise Benefits

This exercise increases flexibility of the gastrocnemius, and it is a good runner's stretch.

Hints for Various Age Levels

Stress trying to press heel to floor.

Assessment

The assessment form for this exercise appears as a full-size form for easy printing on the bound-in CD-ROM at the back of this book.

Child's Pose

Vocabulary

- deltoids
- triceps

Instructions

1. Starting position: Kneel behind the ball on both knees, with hands on ball and tops of feet touching the floor (toes not tucked under) (see figure 10.14a).
2. With arms extended, roll the ball away as far as possible until back is level with the floor or until tension is felt in back (see figure 10.14b).
3. Keep arms straight, and press head toward floor (see figure 10.14c).
4. Pull back until seated on heels (see figure 10.14d).

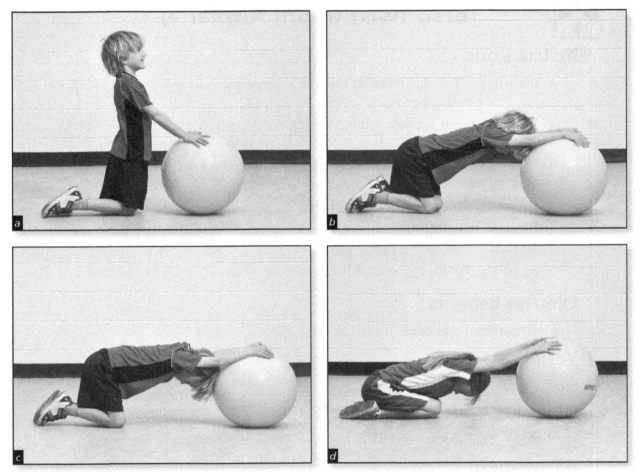

Figure 10.14 Child's Pose: *(a)* starting position; *(b)* rolling ball away; *(c)* pressing head toward floor; *(d)* pulling back until seated on heels.

(continued)

Child's Pose   *(continued)*

Exercise Benefits

This exercise stretches the shoulders (**deltoids**), upper back (trapezius), and arms (**triceps**).

Hints for Various Age Levels

This stretch feels marvelous and is often the finish of a work-out.

Assessment

The assessment form for this exercise appears as a full-size form for easy printing on the bound-in CD-ROM at the back of this book.

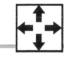

Torso Twist (From Airplane)

Instructions

1. Starting position: Lie prone on the ball, legs extended, arms out to sides in the airplane position (see figure 10.15*a*).
2. Place one hand on floor while twisting trunk as far as possible (see figure 10.15*b*).
3. Ideally, the arms are at a 180-degree angle between floor and ceiling (see figure 10.15*c*).
4. Keep feet on floor, and twist from hips not ankles.
5. If comfortable, continue to turn until chest is open to the ceiling (see figure 10.15*d*).
6. Reverse the twist, and stretch in opposite direction.

Exercise Benefits

This exercise increases flexibility in the spine, back, and chest.

Variations

See Torso Turners on page 58 in chapter 6.

Hints for Various Age Levels

Move slowly until comfortable with this stretch. It is very powerful.

Assessment

The assessment form for this exercise appears as a full-size form for easy printing on the bound-in CD-ROM at the back of this book.

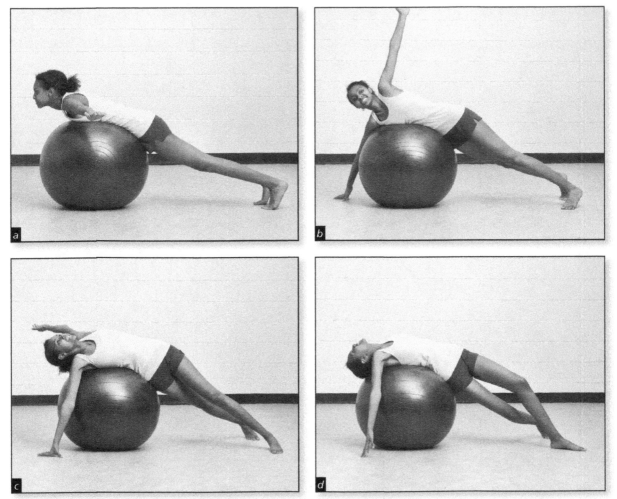

Figure 10.15 Torso Twist: *(a)* starting position; *(b)* twisting the trunk; *(c)* arms at 180-degree angle; *(d)* chest open to ceiling.

PART III

Exercise Balls, Active Seating Devices, and Sensory Baskets: From Brain Research to Balancing Our Lives at Home and Work

In part III, we offer suggestions for the use of exercise balls, active seating devices, and sensory baskets in the classroom, at work, and at home. Chapter 11 discusses brain research and the great benefits you'll derive from using the ball and modifying your lifestyle. Chapter 12 includes some information about using the ball to teach fitness at all levels. In writing chapter 13, we worked closely with classroom teachers and students to develop detailed descriptions and discussion on the use of balls, active seating devices, and sensory baskets in the classroom. We're hoping it will inspire more teachers to include these items in their classrooms. Chapter 14 presents ideas on adding exercise balls, active seating devices, and sensory integration into your home and work environments. We include party suggestions and ideas that you won't want to miss.

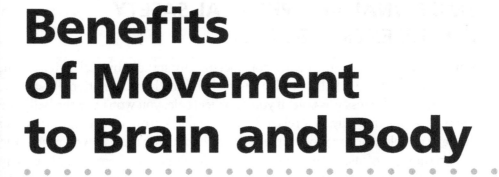

eleven

Benefits of Movement to Brain and Body

· ·

We have a great deal of interest in how brain research pertains to people of all ages, demonstrating the relationship between daily movement and brain functioning. The complexity of brain functioning offers a challenge when teaching new skills and tasks to a diverse group of learners in the same way it is a challenge for each learner. Hopefully, we all learn from our daily interactions with the physical world and all of its inhabitants.

We include physical and emotional safety in this chapter because lots of things happen in our brains when we are trying out new physical activities, and we want your experiences on the exercise ball to be positive and productive. In addition to physical and emotional safety, this chapter also discusses the three Ns (neurobiology, neurogenesis, and neuroplasticity); attention-deficit disorder and attention-deficit/ hyperactivity disorder (ADD and ADHD); and the effects of exercise on your brain to help you understand the critical importance of movement and exercise to learning and daily life.

There has been a strong, steady flow of research on the brain and how it functions. Brain imaging has expanded, and a variety of brain-scanning techniques are available (Sousa 2006). Brain imaging or brain scanning is a way for scientists to look at the structures and workings of the brain. At the current time, the available imaging and scanning technologies are

- EEG (electroencephalography),
- CAT (computerized axial tomography) scans,
- PET (positron emission tomography) scans,
- MRI and fMRI (magnetic resonance imaging and functional magnetic resonance imaging) machines, and
- MEG (magnetoencephalography).

Researchers can actually see how the brain functions and responds to different stimuli (Healy 2004). Some of the research lays out suggestions for helping all of us be our most productive selves (Kay 2000).

EMOTIONAL AND PHYSICAL SAFETY ON THE EXERCISE BALLS

Your comfort level is critical when considering any sort of physical activity. Whenever you are using exercise balls, you have to feel physically and emotionally safe, with the least amount of stress possible. If you don't feel safe, you won't use the ball. The brain reacts in a positive way to a relaxed, comfortable setting (Jensen 2000). Often, it is the very people who are most apprehensive about using the ball who need it the most.

The thought of using the ball may scare some people. Some people may just not consider themselves the athletic type. When people grow up without successful experiences in physical education, sports, and athletics, they tend not to be adventurous in the physical world. This can lead to inactivity and a fear of things related to physical activity. If you are a fitness trainer, therapist, or teacher, it's important to keep this in mind when working with people on the ball. Being sensitive and taking steps to be sure people are at ease emotionally and physically when using the exercise ball will be critical to your success. If you are a first-time user and have some fears about using the ball, you may want to work with an expert when getting started.

When teaching a large group to work with exercise balls, some people will need extra help, and you'll want to get the other people working safely and independently in order to be able to work with those who need more assistance. I (Anne) recently worked with a new student who had a physical disability. He had serious balance and coordination issues that appeared not to have been addressed in the past. He was scared of the ball, and I knew it was going to take time to get him comfortable on the ball. First, I gave him a ball that was slightly deflated, which makes it easier to balance on. Next, I simplified the activities and with his permission physically assisted him. Finally, I showed him modifications he could make while using the ball. It did not take long for him to start smiling. He told me that no one had ever helped him learn physical things before, and he thought this was really fun! It was fun because I made him feel safe in this novel situation. My modifications and suggestions included the following:

- Using a larger ball that was somewhat deflated
- Moving very slowly
- Going back to an easier exercise, or movement, when things got too challenging

Fitness centers and school gymnasiums are often filled to capacity with people of varying skill abilities and needs. In our teaching experience, it has not always been easy to get extra help for those who need it in fitness centers and schools. This sometimes leads those people who need help to drop out. It may take extra time and energy, but you must work with those who have not had a lot of experience or success in movement settings because they are the very people who most need the exercises to improve strength and balance. When people are comfortable and successful while using the exercise ball, and use it regularly, they can improve their balance and core strength. This can lead to a reduction in accidental falls. Improving balance and core strength are two of the greatest benefits of using the exercise ball.

THE THREE NS: NEUROBIOLOGY, NEUROGENESIS, AND NEUROPLASTICITY

The three Ns are neurobiology, neurogenesis, and neuroplasticity. **Neurobiology** is the study of the nervous system's cells (soma) and the way these cells are organized into functional circuits that process information and modify or alter behavior (Schwartz 2003). One area neurobiologists study is neurogenesis. In investigating neurogenesis, scientists have learned new information about neuroplasticity. This section explains the importance of neurogenesis and neuroplasticity to learning.

Neurogenesis is the creation of new neural cells (Ratey 2001). Originally, neuroscientists thought neurogenesis occurred only in newborns, and that the brain was hardwired once fully developed—generally considered by adolescence (Ratey 2008). Scientists now have evidence that neurogenesis also occurs in adults (Schwartz 2003). This is why neuroplasticity is important.

Neuroplasticity refers to changes in the brain as a result of experience and especially movement. Scientists have found that the brain continues to be rewired throughout life. In fact, change occurs in both the structure and function of neurons. A key aspect of neuroplasticity is the importance of the enviroment. Moving, thinking, and learning are critical to this rewiring. Novel experiences are especially important (Ratey 2008). Interacting with an exercise ball counts as a novel experience that ignites neuroplasticity and alters our brain functioning.

ATTENTION-DEFICIT DISORDER AND ATTENTION-DEFICIT/HYPERACTIVITY DISORDER

Attention-deficit disorder and attention-deficit/hyperactivity disorder (ADD/ADHD) are disorders that some experts consider more of traits when the person involved is able to function with no inhibition of work and social life. The label of having ADD/ADHD can be misleading because people who have symptoms of ADD/ADHD actually hyperfocus (long-lasting concentration on one thing) when they are in an environment that most suits *their needs and interests* (Hallowell and Ratey 1995). ADD/ADHD is more of a *fluctuation in focus than a deficit*. When the environment is not working for a person with ADD/ADHD, it can be very hard on that person as well as those around him (Hallowell and Ratey 1995). There are wonderful books available that break down the complex spectrum of ADD/ADHD and show how to make life easier for everyone involved. Thankfully, many of the books are also available in CD format for those who respond better when listening than reading. My favorite books on the subject are listed in the resource section of this book.

One way to help people with ADD/ADHD is to use an exercise ball or other modification (FitBall Seating Disc, FitBall Wedge, FitBall Air Cushion) when sitting in a chair for extended periods of time is required. ADD/ADHD has a spectrum of variables that surface as characteristics of the disorder. The inability to sit still for a long time in one position or place can be especially bothersome in some settings where people's work can be disturbed by another person's constant movement and fidgeting. The amount of time spent sitting before the fidgeting starts often depends on the activity being performed and the topic being read or written about.

Exercise balls and alternative movement devices for chairs have different effects on different people. We have spent time working with classroom teachers, physical therapists, occupational therapists, and psychologists in an attempt to integrate exercise balls and alternative movement devices for chairs into the classrooms and home environments of students with ADD/ADHD and other challenging issues. Recently I've been experimenting with wedges, discs, and cushions that fit into chairs for settings where people are not ready for the balls. I'm seeing lots of success with different students who had been struggling with a variety of distractability issues.

When working in schools we usually discuss a plan for the classroom, students, and teacher. This plan can include the classroom and other learning environments. It is an individualized plan for those who are having problems functioning in the classroom as a result of having ADD/ADHD or distractibility issues. In an effort not to single out a student who is struggling, we frequently suggest that several balls or alternative cushions be made available in classrooms. It is important to note that balls and cushions will benefit the user for reasons other than ADD/ADHD or distractability. A desire to maintain or improve muscle tone and core strength are two other good reasons a person would want to use alternative seating. You can read more about integrating balls into the classroom in chapter 13 of this book.

In all of his books, John Ratey informs us of the need for regular movement and exercise. He states that all people have a certain degree of attention problems and that everyone can benefit from moving, not just people diagnosed with ADHD (Ratey 2008). Hannaford, who believes if she were in school now she would be seen as having ADHD because of her constant need to move in order to learn, concurs with the need for movement to enhance learning (Hannaford 1995). As early as 1994, schools were experimenting with using balls as chairs (Illi 1994). Sitting on the ball allows movement that enables people with ADHD to keep their bodies and brains focused.

YOUR BRAIN ON EXERCISE

Movement is transformative—it enhances brainpower and helps you think better and be smarter (Jensen 1996). Activity brings additional oxygen-carrying blood to the brain, thereby improving processing. At work or in a teaching–learning environment, people can think and learn more efficiently and effectively if they take frequent movement breaks. After 20 minutes of inactive sitting, blood pools in the seat and feet (Sousa 2006). Movement recirculates that blood. Integrating movement increases productivity and learning. Examples of integrating movement in a workplace include stepping away from the computer and walking while talking with a coworker; walking down the hall instead of sending an e-mail; and having a small group of coworkers walk and discuss issues of concern. Examples of integrating movement and learning in a school environment include walking and talking with a partner or small group about the three most important things you just learned; walking and touching four things in the room that are oval shapes; and standing and presenting what you think was important about the lesson you just covered to the person next to you. More movement examples for learning and productivity appear in chapter 13.

Movement on a regular basis is what keeps the brain awake, engaged, and literally growing (Ratey 2008). When people are in the right environment, they can actually undergo neural rewiring and brain growth. Novelty experiences are especially beneficial to keep the brain active. Even though I've been living with a large pearl-colored ball in my house for many years, it's still a novelty and an attraction. I use it in a variety of ways. Sometimes I sit on it, other times I stretch out my back or do some core strength exercises on it. The ball as I use it in my house is a piece of furniture and a piece of exercise equipment. It's an integral part of my home, and it helps me stay focused and improves my balance, core strength, and flexibility.

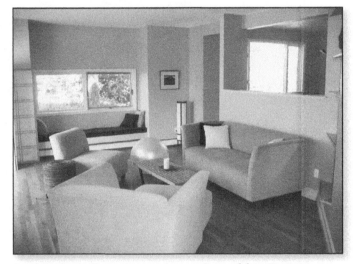

An exercise ball can be used as a piece of furniture or a piece of exercise equipment in a living room.

© Anne Spalding

SUMMARY

Physical and emotional safety is primary when using the exercise ball. Brain research has clearly shown the importance of the three Ns—neurobiology, neurogenesis, and neuroplasticity—to learning. People who have ADD/ADHD can benefit from the movement provided by the exercise ball. Movement is essential to the process of learning, and increasing your daily movement is essential for increasing brainpower. You will think better, improve processing, and learn more efficiently when you incorporate the exercise ball in your daily activities.

twelve

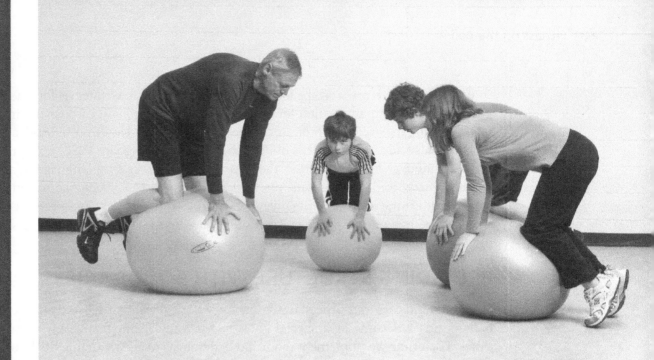

Strategies for Teaching With the Exercise Ball

· ·

Teaching can be exhilarating and exhausting. From the very young to the very old, each of us is physically and emotionally different. As teachers, instructors, therapists, and trainers, we must see our students or clients for the unique individuals they are, from one day to the next. For those of us who work with 20 or more people at a time, this is no small feat.

As diverse as we all are, there are also many similarities between people, both young and old. Many characteristics remain clear and recognizable from 5 to 85 and beyond. From the fearful, shy, and timid to the bold, daredevilish, and ornery, each individual needs to be acknowledged and appreciated. Effective strategies need to be used when teaching physical activities so that all participants progress toward active, healthy lifestyles. This chapter discusses ways to meet students and clients where they are in terms of behaviors and characteristics, to celebrate the diverse and unique, and, finally, to find ways to help everyone feel successful.

We'd like to give you a recipe for customizing your various strategies for teaching. We'll start with our suggestion for establishing boundaries and discuss the importance of using the overhead projector, projection system, and large posters as learning tools. We also address the needs of English as a second language (ESL) learners and English language learners (ELLs); the importance of integrating language, reading, writing, math, and science with physical activities; and why practice to reinforce correct patterning is critical. Finally, we explain learning centers and projects using the exercise ball and how exercise balls are being used in one specific high school physical education class.

PROVIDING STRUCTURE WITH BOUNDARIES

Setting boundaries and procedures is the most critical element when using exercise balls. Linda has come as a special guest to teach my (Anne's) students numerous times. Each time we implement more and better ideas to clearly define the boundaries and procedures for using exercise balls in the gymnasium. It is always best to start off firm and structured with the boundaries and procedures and then back off a little later, if or when it seems appropriate. Skill acquisition requires repetition of correctly performed movements. Practice makes permanent, and if your students or clients don't learn the benefits of correct form and mechanics from the beginning, they may miss out on the benefits or possibly injure themselves or others.

Suggested boundaries include the following:

- Treat the ball as an exercise or therapeutic tool rather than a toy.
- Be respectful of other people's working space in order to be safe.
- *Never* push the ball from underneath another person.

INTEGRATING LANGUAGE, READING, WRITING, MATH, AND SCIENCE INTO PHYSICAL ACTIVITY SETTINGS

As teachers we are in the driver's seat. The word choices we make affect our students. ESL or ELL students and native English speakers are constantly learning new words from us. We can play more with our words and make learning fun and meaningful while increasing everyone's active vocabulary. People of all ages enjoy rhymes and an occasional play on words. Language is fun, and once you start to play with it, it can take on a life of its own. Learning new words—both abstract and concrete—helps your brain stay healthy by keeping it engaged. Abstract words, such as *space*, *time*, and *force*, require concrete examples and images in order to be fully understood and integrated into our daily lives (Sousa 2005). Teaching the concept of force, for example, can be accompanied by visual aids and overheads. Furthermore, using a physical lesson with the exercise ball can drive home the message of this abstract concept.

Here is an example of guiding a person on the ball using the concept of force:

- While sitting in the center of the ball, use a light force to initiate a bounce.
- While keeping your bottom on the ball, explore using light, medium, and strong force to bounce safely.

• Ask participants to feel the changes in force and to discuss the experience by having them pair and share their discoveries about the concept of force while bouncing on the ball.

There doesn't need to be anything contrived or forced about integrating reading, writing, math, and science into our physical education programs. Taking a little more time and energy to pull out a book with great anatomy illustrations or sharing a rhyme or poem on the overhead can really spark students' interest and motivate them to explore a wide variety of subjects. Often the light will come on when people see and feel the connections between physical movement and science, math, and reading concepts. Combining verbal-based information, image-based information, and movement-based information has positive implications for instruction.

Learning is constant. When Linda visits my school, Crest View Elementary, to teach with me, I always share with my students that she has a PhD in fitness and how much I always learn from her. I refer to her as the fitness expert when she's not at school. The big picture of lifelong fitness includes the following topics: eating healthy foods, staying hydrated, and participating in different types of physical activities. Don't underestimate your potential influence on your students and clients. Linda has had former students approach her, years after learning about the importance of staying hydrated throughout the day, and pull out their water bottles to show her that the healthy habit she taught them in elementary school stuck with them.

USING OVERHEADS PROJECTORS

We are big advocates of using overhead projectors or projection systems in all teaching–learning settings. After using them for professional conferences, we started using them more in our gymnasiums. Using projection systems really gets people's attention and keeps them focused and on task. As the saying goes, a picture is worth a thousand words. A good illustration can help the class see the exact body position and mechanics of a movement or exercise. We include clear and detailed illustrations and photos in this book and on the bound-in CD-ROM because we know that when using visual aids, you can reach and teach your group while freeing yourself up to assist those who need extra help with the movements or exercises.

Organizing Overheads

Over the course of time, I (Anne) have come to more fully understand my need for organizational strategies when I use a traditional, old-fashioned overhead projector. I've fine-tuned and changed my overhead strategies for efficiency. My current favorite organizational strategy is to get large pieces of colored paper and lay out the paper either on tables or on the floor. The colors are my cue as to what category of overhead is on the sheet—flexibility is yellow, strength is orange, and cardiorespiratory is red (for the heart!). This helps me choose efficiently the category and exercise I want to address.

My schedule currently does not give me any time in between different age groups of students. I'll have a class of fifth-grade students followed immediately by kindergarten students. That means I need to have a wide variety of overheads ready to quickly show appropriate progressions according to the grade level and the students.

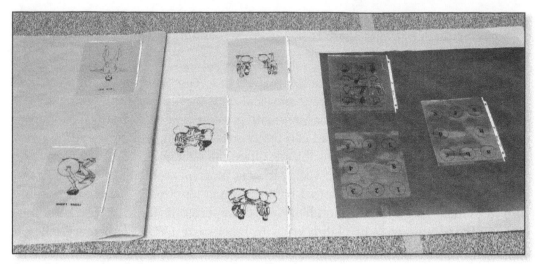

Organizing overheads for a projector using colored paper.

I try to customize the exercises to meet the needs of each group. Experimenting with different combinations of ball exercises keeps classes fun and engaging. Sequences of different exercises allow students to remember three to seven specific moves that they will be able to perform on cue in small or large groups. I teach these sequences in chunks so the students can recall the order of the exercises. I may choose a few exercises in which participants are sitting and bouncing on the ball, followed by some balance, strength, and flexibility exercises.

As Linda, my mother, and I took photos for the preliminary planning and writing of this book, I started using the photos on my laptop computer with a projector—a little more modern system. This has been very efficient and effective in the gymnasium. Linda's two kids, Lizzy and Michael, were our models, and we have some exercises in which they did a move on the right and then the left side of the body. We quickly discovered that if you moved back and forth from slide to slide it looked animated, as if they were kicking their legs in the air. This strategy was a big hit and has kept my students very focused. Don't forget that all the photos that appear in this book are found on your bound-in CD-ROM, so be sure to make good use of them on your computer.

Teaching ESL Students and ELLs Using Overheads

Overheads and posters are also great for your ESL students and ELLs. Illustrations along with demonstrations can get any group of learners on board quickly. The ESL and ELL group will benefit from clear and concise directional words, clues, and cues, especially when they are used in conjunction with photos or illustrations. It uses the "show, tell, do" method, and the words make sense and have meaning. Always show and tell slowly enough to allow the students to adequately absorb the new information and to be sure it sticks with them. When learning a new language, repetition is very important, and less is more in terms of word choices. The consistent use of concise cue words allows everyone to be able to perform the exercises without always looking at the pictures or posters on the overhead. This is true for all learners, not just ESL and ELL groups. See! Say! Do!

USING THE PEER TEACHER, TUTOR, AND COACH STRATEGY

It's tough to teach a large group by yourself. Getting the class on board as teachers, tutors, and coaches is a quick way to successful teaching. I've discussed this with my students, and a class of mine brought me a homemade sign, "All students are both teachers and learners." It's posted on the door for students to see as they enter the gym. It is very empowering to have students help each other. I've added this new poster I made as another reminder in the classroom.

All Students Are

- Learners
- Coaches
- Teachers

Often our groups have people who can easily turn and help their neighbor, and it's a very positive social interaction. Don't forget to do the pair-and-share activities introduced in chapter 3 and more defined in chapter 4. To review and give an example of the method for doing pair-and-share activities, have everyone in the class pair up and ask each other the following questions when doing an exercise:

- What did you learn? (The specific clue, cue, or category of an exercise.)
- Why is it important? (Some possibilities include building strength, increasing your heart rate, and improving flexibility.)
- How can you use it in your life? (Can you do this exercise in any other settings? Do you need to have a ball to do it? Could you do it without a ball when you don't have one with you?)

The learning process is much more powerful when the learner is invited to discuss the topic as opposed to the teacher summarizing. Pair and share is a great way to develop ownership in the learning environment.

SHARING THE ODOMETER ANALOGY

Whenever I try to explain to my classes that the more time they spend on the ball or correctly practicing any skill, the easier it will become, I share with them this analogy:

When you first get your driver's license, you haven't had much time on the road. Some driving programs have new drivers document the time they spend driving behind the wheel with an adult in the car. Some states also have a new graduated license program. To avoid distractions when you first receive a driver's license, you are not allowed to drive at night or have other young people in the car with you until you have spent lots of time driving behind the wheel to improve your driving skills and performance.

An odometer is a mechanism that keeps track of the number of miles or kilometers a vehicle has been driven. If you haven't seen an odometer, then your homework is to ask if you can see the odometer in the car the next time you are getting a ride somewhere.

For every mile the car is driven, another mile is recorded on the odometer. It's fun to find out the distance between places you travel by checking in with the driver to see the distance traveled.

Good athletes spend time performing their favorite skills (e.g., shooting baskets or hitting baseballs or golf balls). Whenever you spend time improving your skills or improving your fitness level, you can think about your internal odometer. Remember that the skill or exercise needs to be done correctly because practice makes permanent, or at least makes it extremely hard to change. Have you heard the old saying, "You can't teach an old dog new tricks"? Well, there is some truth to it, and it's really hard to break habits if you've learned a skill incorrectly.

I check in with students in all different skill areas, such as jump rope, especially when they are trying to learn to turn and jump double-Dutch ropes. They really get the odometer theory now, they know it's going to take time to learn new skills and activities, and they understand what a learning curve is. Those "got it" moments are so sweet, and the only way we can get there is if we persevere.

CREATING LEARNING CENTERS

While using overheads or posters, we are able to get our larger groups on the ball. If you don't have enough balls for everyone, or if you are ready for another way to use the balls, you can create learning centers. If you have only four to six balls, you can set up a learning center of balls combined with other skills or fitness centers. If you've purchased enough balls for an entire class, you could design learning centers where they are all active and engaged with different skills and fitness concepts in different parts of the room. However, you want to organize the learning environment so you'll be able to use your posters or overheads to keep the group focused on the specific exercises you want them to learn or practice.

As time goes by, you may want to let your class choose their favorite exercises and organize the lesson in such a way that advanced learners will put together sequences or routines to teach others. This can take on a life of its own because once students are motivated, they will want to create and share with others.

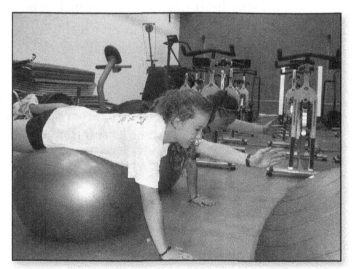

Boulder High School students using exercise balls as a learning center.
© Anne Spalding

MAKING MOVIES AND COMMERCIALS

This year I had the chance to use a new DVD camera and portable viewer to enrich and enhance learning experiences. Letting students know they can be recorded when a sequence or routine is done well and ready to share with others is a powerful tool. Once you have a good demonstration on the DVD, show the others and watch how the excitement grows. You will then have a recording that can be used to teach other classes or be shared in a center to keep things lively and on task.

Commercials that advertise fitness are the next step. After focusing on fitness concepts, it is very educational for students to write and perform advertisements. You'll need the following:

- Visual aids such as models and posters of the human body systems
- Exercise balls and other equipment such as jump ropes, resistance bands, or light hand weights
- Rubrics of requirements and grading criteria for the fitness commercials

Again, once you have videotaped or made DVDs of students' work, you can use them both to teach and inspire your other students.

INTEGRATING EXERCISE BALLS IN THE GYMNASIUM: A SAMPLE HIGH SCHOOL PROGRAM

While we were writing this book, I contacted Monique Guidry, a physical education teacher of 20 years plus who teaches at Boulder High School in Colorado. I gave her some information from our first book and shared our thoughts on including people of all ages in our second book.

Ms. Guidry had recently purchased some exercise balls and had a new cardiorespiratory exercise room with stationary bikes and treadmills directly adjacent to a mat room. When we met she was in the process of planning a winter fitness class. She thought the combination of the cardio room with a core strength class using mat exercises and balls to emphasize core strength would be a good fit.

Ms. Guidry used a book containing exercises on the mats that emphasize deliberate slowness and use the word *prehabilitation*. I thought it was a match made in heaven when she shared this with me. Linda and I have always discussed using the exercise balls as a way of preventing injuries in the first place by increasing balance, coordination, core strength, and flexibility.

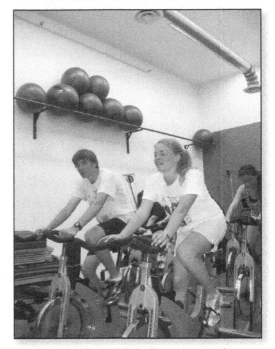

Stationary bikes with ball storage in the background.
© Anne Spalding

Organizing a New Program

Ms. Guidry separated her classes into two groups, purple and gold, representing the high school colors. When students arrived, they were to dress out and then let her know they were present. She placed a dot by their names, and they went directly to an assigned area—either the cardio room or the mat and exercise ball room, and got started on their assigned routines. They would spend 20 minutes in each area.

Cardio was spent on the treadmills and stationary bikes, while the mat room emphasized strength in the neck to midback area with a focus on balance, coordination, stabilizing strength, and flexibility using the mats and exercise balls. The students did sets of repetitions for each exercise.

Some Specific Thoughts From Ms. Guidry on Using Exercise Balls

Ms. Guidry and her students were intrigued by the sense of play on the ball. She made a point of sharing with them how awkward the ball exercises would feel when they were first trying them out. She made it lighthearted so that students did not feel too self-conscious about the time it can take to perform the exercises correctly in front of others. The positions were not always easy to assume, and she liked the way the students had to pay so much attention to themselves and their own body position. This kept them focused on the exercise instead of others.

Using verbal cues was critical. Ms. Guidry used a notebook with the exercises in it. She kept the verbal cues concise, using "Belly on the center of the ball" and the letters Y, T, W, and L for arm and leg shapes. Other favorite cues were "Elbows up," "Squeeze shoulders," and "Fists on the floor." She had one blind student in her class, whom she partnered up with a practicum student. If the practicum student wasn't available, she would pair this student up with a classmate. She kept her cues concise and easy to visualize.

Mondays were the hardest, as that was the day she taught new exercises each week, and she noticed the students were particularly observant, looking at her for the visual clues. By Tuesday she shared that they were less dependent on her and moved along more quickly. At the end of the week, she handed over the exercise notebook to her students and had partners lead each other through the exercises. She believed her strong cues and language carried over, and students picked up the exercises and were able to perform them comfortably.

As the class progressed and the students' fitness levels and comfort on the balls improved, Ms. Guidry gradually introduced more difficult exercises. This was a winter fitness class, and she believed that, for this time of the year, the balls were key in spicing up the fitness program. We discussed the fact that when this book comes out, she will have a lot more illustrated exercises she can use as handheld visuals, posters, or overheads. Be sure to use the CD-ROM in the back of this book to create your own handheld visuals, posters, overheads, and slide shows on your computer.

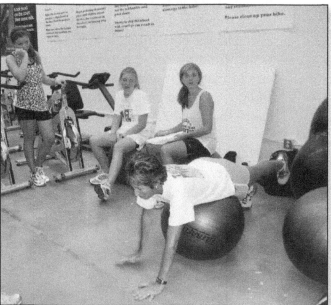

Ms. Guidry demonstrating on the exercise ball.
© Anne Spalding

SUMMARY

We hope this chapter has given you ideas for effectively using the exercise balls. By setting boundaries; thinking more about integrating language, science, and math; and making good use of visuals you should have a recipe for success. Using participants as teachers and coaches has helped us give individualized attention to those who need it and keeps everyone in our classes on the ball. We also think your group will enjoy the concept of centers and projects. Finally, it is our hope that Ms. Guidry from Boulder High School inspires the integration of exercise balls in fitness classes with other equipment, such as stationary bikes, and that you are ready to either start using exercise balls or expand your existing program. In chapter 13, we'll share ideas for integrating the exercise balls and other more active sitting options into classroom settings.

thirteen

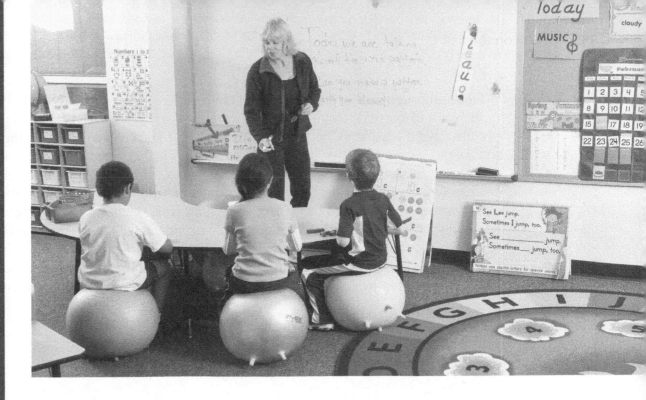

Using Exercise Balls, Active Seating Options, and Sensory Integration Ideas in Classroom Settings

● ●

If God would have known what schools would be like, he would have made kids differently.—Albert Einstein

I (Anne) have been a teacher now for more than 25 years, and in those years the job has not become easier. Actually, it's become harder—much harder. I believe the reason it's gotten harder relates to the saying that "the more you know, the more you know that you don't know." Between Linda and me, we've accumulated well over 50 years of experience. Right now there is so much research being done on the brain that my own brain is swimming in it, and I'm more determined than ever to advocate for meeting the needs of all kids and people whose lives seem a little too challenging.

Educating our uniquely diverse children is one of the greatest challenges of our time, and none of us can do it alone. We have to be able to talk about the issues and not be embarrassed or ashamed of things that may have been taboo to talk about in the past.

In this chapter, we discuss the use of exercise balls in the classroom to help students with special needs, but that's not all we're going to talk about. We're going to talk about **sensory integration**: the ability to integrate or bring together all the information that comes to us through our senses (seeing, hearing, smelling, and feeling). We'll discuss bringing other active seating alternatives into the classroom. Linda and I have both introduced the use of exercise balls in various classrooms and schools. In this chapter we give you thoughts, guidelines, and suggestions for using exercise balls in classroom settings as well as information on active seating alternatives, including

- FitBall Seating Discs,
- FitBall Wedges,
- FitBall Air Cushions, and
- Movin'Sit Air Cushions.

These are all air filled and can be used on the floor or added to any furniture used for sitting, including wheelchairs. They are used to improve posture, strengthen the core of your body, and increase movement while seated.

We'll discuss something I've been playing with and talking about with physical therapists (PTs) and occupational therapists (OTs) for years—sensory baskets, the concept of regulatory items and equipment to give suggestions and choices to teachers and students about how to regulate their way through the day and to customize their own "motion promotion."

At the end of this chapter, we share some survey results and quotes from both teachers and students in regard to using exercise balls and other active seating options while in a classroom. We hope this feedback will give you a feel for how others have integrated exercise balls and active seating options into their classrooms.

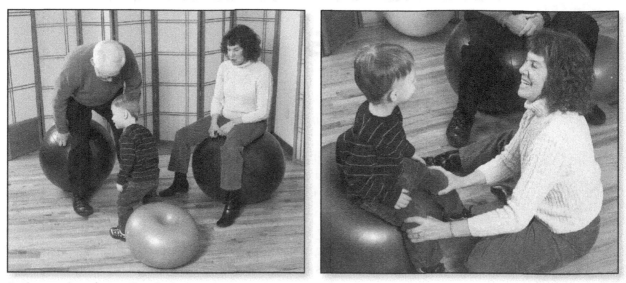

Active seating alternatives include a donut seat.

NOBODY'S PERFECT

Don't panic when you start to read this story. I got permission from my mom to tell it. It was time for me to start first grade, and my mom said she parked the car in front of the school, leaving me in it to wait for her. It was common practice back then to leave kids unattended in the car while you went in somewhere to do something. So, mom went in and completed the appropriate paperwork to sign me up in the Catholic school where my sisters were already enrolled. My sisters, by the way, were and are extremely well behaved, and both are really smart. So, by contrast, signing up the wild child (that's me) must have been a little scary for my mom. She told me that when she completed the paperwork, they asked if there was anything else they needed to know about her youngest daughter, who would be starting first grade soon. She said no. Then she came and got in the car, looked at me, and marched right back into the building and told them I had lost my eye but that I wouldn't be any trouble, or something like that. It strikes me as extremely funny now, and I want to say, "Gosh, I hope you all can find it." (The eye, that is. Sorry, comic relief.) I'm telling this story as a very personal icebreaker, and believe me, those are important when talking to people about the special needs of their children, especially as it relates to education.

Every child in every classroom is someone's baby. Our greatest hopes and dreams rest in those little bundles of joy. Wow, that's a tough spot to be in, and now you're going to tell someone that his or her child is less than perfect. I'm sorry, but that's a tough pill for anyone to swallow. If our kids are not perfect—and let's face it, nobody is perfect—it may take time to come to grips with this new perception. Whatever it is that is perceived as a little askew can make aspects of school and life more challenging. We may even end up in denial. Yes, that's right. I love you, Mom, and every other mom and dad out there who has to come to grips with the fact that their child is perceived as less than perfect. Any way you look at it, this topic is extremely difficult to discuss.

We can't leave the political side of education out of the discussion. It is important to understand the language that educators use regularly to describe programs, policies, and students so you can be an informed advocate.

Following are some of the acronyms that educators use:

- NCLB, or No Child Left Behind
- AYP, or annual yearly progress
- RTI, or response to intervention

You think *you're* confused, educators have to learn this educational jargon all the time. Now for the quiz:

1. What is NCLB?
2. What is AYP?
3. What is an RTI?

How did you do? Did you look back to see if your guess was correct? Good for you; that's the idea of taking in small bits of information that make sense and have meaning. Now, pair and share with another person (refer to chapter 4 for details). Did the information stick with you?

Now, what does NCLB mean? It's a government-mandated policy that all public school children are to be proficient in content areas. AYP means that public schools meet yearly prescribed goals. An RTI consists of data-driven strategies to meet the needs of struggling learners.

That's where we are in public education right now at the beginning of 2009. As an educator looking toward the challenges we face now and in the future, I'm exhilarated, energized, exhausted, and scared. Today more people are talking about things that make learning difficult and how to intervene to make learning easier. RTIs are supposed to make it easier on the kids and the teachers and help us all move into the future more balanced: academically, physically, and emotionally. That's right, I use the word emotional because I'm no longer scared of it. I've read enough evidence that without a relaxed emotional state, none of us can perform academically or physically. I've ridden the roller coaster of emotions and it makes me a little dizzy to look back on where I was and where I am right now.

I'm writing this book from a place where I spent years in classrooms, which included well over 30 students, in the back of the room in literally the last seat in the last row. I was looking out of one eye and having a heck of a time focusing on anything since I certainly couldn't see the blackboard. I had a brain that was dancing and a body that wanted to move all the time, whether because of my need to move or possibly ADD, but I had to sit in a hard chair and pretty much not talk.

Not being allowed to talk used to kill me, and I'll share a quick story of the disastrous results of one of my talking episodes: I was put out in the hall for talking. I was scared to death because that really was the last straw, especially for a girl in this school where we all wore plaid uniforms and white blouses every day for eight years. If you were in the hall and someone saw you there, it was huge. So there I was, heart racing, and I see Mrs. Fulkerson, my mom's friend who worked in the cafeteria, walking toward me. I recall the moment and my reaction vividly: With a big smile I said, "Hello, Mrs. Fulkerson. I'm out here because I'm so far ahead in reading." Mrs. Fulkerson smiled sweetly and kept walking.

My history and my stories are exactly what give me the credibility to write this book and this chapter. This writing thing is a bear for me, by the way. I've experienced some trauma in my life, as many of us have. Repeated surgical procedures from the age of three on have really impacted me. In fact some of the doctors that I have worked with have mentioned that I have Post Traumatic Stress Disorder (PTSD)-like symptoms. These symptoms may actually be the root cause of my ADD like symptoms. "Co-Occurring" conditions are exactly what make regulating your way through the day so critical.

Think of PTSD and ADD as a spectrum of behaviors. It's more of a way of being and operating than a diagnosis or an identity. It requires some rethinking in the way that people operate and can look different from day to day, emotion to emotion, person to person, and situation to situation.

I'm celebrating brain-based classrooms that honor peoples' needs to move and talk to learn. I'm advocating for active seating options, such as exercise balls, wedges, and discs, and sensory baskets—which I'll describe in more detail later in the chapter—to help people regulate their way through the day.

When researching this chapter, I was told about a wonderful book, *Uniquely Gifted: Identifying and Meeting the Needs of the Twice-Exceptional Student*. Forty-eight different experts contributed to this book, which is edited by Kiesa Kay. The list of contributors includes John J. Ratey, MD; Howard Gardner, PhD; and Rebecca Hutchins, OD, FCOVD, who is my eye doctor. The book was extremely enlightening because I had not read very much about students who are talented and gifted (TAG) and have some type of disability on top of their giftedness. This book was enjoyable, yet painful, to read at times because of the firsthand stories about children and their families struggling to get appropriate educational services. It also made me recall that my own loving parents took me to the administration center of our local public school system to take a test that I now know was an IQ test, because I'm sure they were scared when I wasn't performing to my potential in the school I was attending. I'm certainly not saying my challenges and frustrations were anyone's fault, because they weren't. However, we now know too much not to speak up and advocate for each other and our dreams of having a happy, productive life where we can make a difference in our communities and the world.

At a time when kids' test scores are published in the newspaper and parents are out shopping for the best school for their children, the pressure for performance is high. The real question should be, how does each of those kids in that classroom learn best? What's their learning style, and what wakes them up and tunes them in so they are available for learning?

SENSORY INTEGRATION

Sensory integration is simply the bringing together of our senses: seeing, hearing, tasting, smelling, and touching. It's something we do naturally all day every day. Each of us sees, hears, tastes, smells, and feels things differently, and for the most part we only know how things look, sound, taste, smell, and feel to us. That's where it gets complicated. When a child is acting a certain way that is terribly annoying, it's not the teacher's fault if she doesn't know that the behavior is actually neurologically or physiologically based. Teachers all over the world are desperately trying to maintain an atmosphere conducive to learning in their classrooms. They are often overwhelmed by the demands of the diverse students in the room at any given moment. In actuality, it's primarily about how each of those students feels physically and emotionally in that room that is the biggest roadblock to learning. It's really about animal instincts and emotions. That's right, we're people and we're animals and we respond to light, heat, sound, and visual stimulation—or the lack of it.

Paying closer attention to our learners and the needs of their senses is perhaps the key to the future improvement of learning environments. World-renowned expert on animal emotions Marc Bekoff (2008) noted in a radio interview that "sensory modalities drive us," and just like wolves, mice, and elephants, humans are physically and emotionally driven by our senses. He mentions in the interview that neurobiologists are calling him about research on animal emotions. Bekoff is hoping that animal research showing parallels between the behaviors and emotions of animals and humans will help the paradigm shift toward more cooperation and compassion in the classroom. Why not start by adding more sensory choices in the classroom? That seems cooperative and compassionate. Students who may function better with additional choices for active seating and other simple, nonintrusive sensory modifications may perk up and be more available for learning.

There are also parallels between emotions and movement and our ancient human history. We used to be hunters and gatherers. Even though most people have stopped moving to gather food and seek safe shelter as in earlier history, there is still an innate need for physical work and movement. Sitting for long periods can be excruciating to some people. Recognizing this innate desire to move may prompt us to make a few changes that engage a student more emotionally and physically.

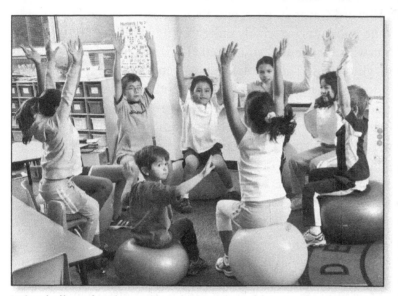

Using balls and active seating devices can add a new fun factor to learning.

Simply adding alternative seating options, sensory integration baskets, and other tools to the classrooms can maximize learning. It could be evolutionary and revolutionary and be proactive rather than reactive to perceived behaviors and academic issues. Maybe it will become more commonplace to see balls, disks, and wedges used as chairs at desks, in reading circles, and in music classes. Just maybe we'll crack things open and start finding ways to adapt and adopt sensory integration ideas that help us regulate our senses to be our happiest, most productive selves. Sold? Great! Now, how do you get started? Read on to find out how to integrate all this good stuff into the classroom.

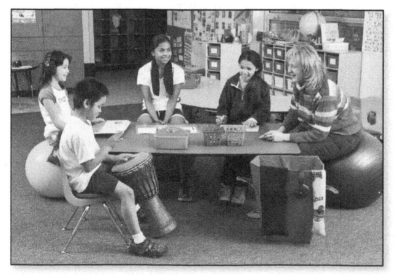

Sensory basket in use in the classroom.

HOW DO I INTRODUCE USING EXERCISE BALLS TO MY STUDENTS?

All teachers are unique, just like the kids they teach, so this is not a one-size-fits-all list of how to introduce exercise balls in your classroom. I've been doing this a long time, and I've arrived at the conclusion that some teachers are eager to use the balls, others desire to use the balls in a limited fashion, and others not at all. I understand and embrace this, and that's why later in this chapter we discuss other alternative seating options such as disks, wedges, and air-filled cushions.

For those who are ready and want to try using exercise balls in your classroom, here are some guidelines:

1. **Reinforce the correct way to sit on the ball** (see figure 5.2*a* on page 41). If a student is going to sit on the ball and get the full benefits and be safe, he needs to see how to do it correctly and practice the correct posture. Some people will not like the ball, and that's okay. Others will like it, but they will be able to sit on the ball with good posture for only a short time at first because they don't have the core strength to maintain the position for very long. That's why choices and options are important.

2. **Start slowly—5 to 10 minutes per student**. Sitting on the ball requires active sitting. It takes muscular strength and endurance. It may be unrealistic to have students sit actively on a ball until they have built up the strength and endurance to not hit the **fatigue zone**. The fatigue zone indicator is slumped posture.

3. **Establish management procedures; taking turns is part of the management.** We have seen good results from one ball for every four people. In our classrooms, we clearly see the need for exercise balls with feet or rubber rings to place the balls on, as necessary, so the balls won't roll when people get up. Without the legs or rubber rings to set them on and keep them in place, the

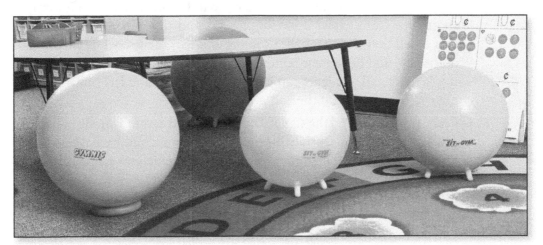

A rubber ring is used to help keep an exercise ball in place.

balls can roll and accidentally be kicked and be a disturbance, a safety hazard, or a distractor factor. Also, providing a storage space for the balls, such as a corner for stacking balls, is important.

4. **Use a small bell as a signal to change ball users.** "Ding," the ball goes to the next person, and nothing needs to be said. Starting with short turns of 5 minutes allows time to build up muscular strength and endurance without hitting the fatigue zone mentioned earlier. A signal can give using the exercise balls a gamelike feeling.

The physical education teacher can play a quiet game of Ball Exchange in physical education class to practice and prepare students to exchange exercise balls in a controlled and quiet way. Ball Exchange can be played as a learning center or with the whole class depending on your needs and the physical education teacher's curriculum and supply of balls. The physical education teacher could add the game to a fitness lesson for the whole class when the balls are already in use. Following are some guidelines for this activity.

1. Start giving directions when all students are sitting correctly on the ball.

2. Inform students that their classroom teacher wants to try using the balls as an alternative to hard chairs. Most students I've worked with are pretty excited by that thought. Tell them that the number of balls in the room can or will vary depending on how well they manage their behavior and the balls as pieces of equipment. If they do well and the teacher is not disturbed by the use of the balls, the balls may become part of the classroom furniture. If the use of the balls is too much work for the classroom teacher or students are not using them safely, they can disappear for an hour, day, week, or forever.

3. Next, tell students that when you ding the bell, or whatever signal you choose to use, they need to calmly and carefully exchange balls with a neighbor close to them. This is one time when the size of the ball doesn't matter too much because the students will be sitting on them for only a short time (see chapter 2 for suggestions and recommendations on getting a ball that fits). If a ball is too big, students can scoot onto the edge of the ball and keep their hands on it to steady the ball and themselves. If it is too small, students can just sit for a second and feel how it's really not that comfortable if the ball is too small.

4. Each time you sound the signal, they slowly and carefully trade balls with a different neighbor. During this time, you can notice and make comments to individuals and the group about positive interactions while the ball is being exchanged.

Some adaptations to this game may include the following:

• Use the Ball Exchange game as a learning center, including anywhere from four to eight students or so, and allow the students to take turns being the teacher and giving the signal to exchange balls. Be sure the students know that they need to make observations of polite, considerate behavior and notice what is happening within the group. That's what good teachers and coaches do: They notice appropriate, efficient, and effective behavior.

- This game could certainly be done in any classroom setting where the teacher is willing to set aside the time and go for it. The only reason we started out with it in the gym is because we're physical education teachers, and that's how we have done it.

Making the Ball Exchange activity a control challenge and reinforcing good transitions with praise can go a long way in establishing clear procedures and expectations for using the exercise balls in your classroom.

5. **Remember that one solution does not fit all.** Some ADD students benefit from short turns on the ball, but they may grow antsy when they have had too much time on the ball. Keep in mind that all people are different on any given day. Be a careful observer for signs that someone is not enjoying or sitting appropriately on the exercise ball. It doesn't need to be a big deal. A simple *That doesn't seem to be working for you today* or *Now you can set the ball in the corner or pass it along to someone else* is sufficient. Empowering people to understand that the beneficial results from sitting on the ball are unique to each person and moment or day is critical to integrating exercise balls into a healthy, active lifestyle.

WHAT ARE THE GUIDELINES FOR USING EXERCISE BALLS IN THE CLASSROOM?

A picture is worth a thousand words, and that is why we suggest having illustrations of the posture for correctly sitting on the ball prominently displayed wherever exercise balls are being used as chairs or stools (see the bound-in CD-ROM for an illustration to use in your classroom). We highly recommend demonstrating the use of the ball, showing the illustrations of proper posture while on the ball, and having students do a pair-and-share activity about the guidelines for using exercise balls before actually using the balls in your room. A review of the following guidelines for using the exercise balls may be necessary if or when you see behaviors and actions that are not up to your behavior management standards:

1. Keep both feet on the floor at all times.
2. Sit in the center of the exercise ball.
3. Use care when sitting down on the ball because exercise balls are very different from a chair.
4. Make sure there are no sharp objects in pockets or on clothing whenever you are around or sitting on the exercise ball.
5. Use hands to steady the ball when getting on or off the ball.
6. Pencils and scissors should always be set on the table when getting on or off the ball.
7. Use small, controlled bounces when seated on the exercise ball. Remember, this is not a toy.
8. Be careful not to kick the ball in the classroom—*ever*.

HOW DO I INTEGRATE THE EXERCISE BALLS INTO THE CLASSROOM?

When integrating exercise balls into their classrooms, some teachers like to start with a couple of balls as a learning center or a reward. I usually give an introduction to using the exercise balls in the classroom in physical education class. This introduction approach seems very beneficial because I have time to tell students how lucky they are that their teacher is willing to try out using the balls in the classroom. I make it very clear that it is a privilege to have the balls in their room. If the balls are not used appropriately, students will lose their privilege to use the ball. This tactic usually works really well. The first time a student is asked to give the ball to another student or set it off to the side, they are disappointed and eager for the next opportunity to show they can use it responsibly.

Cinda Magliolo works at Fireside Elementary in Louisville, Colorado, and this is her second year using exercise balls as chairs. She's very happy with the results she's having, and she sent me this summary of how she uses and organizes the balls in her room.

> *I have two balls per table, and the students simply rotate them clockwise. With this group I had to set some boundaries—feet have to be planted on the floor, which limits the height of their bounce. When they are asking a question or commenting, they must sit still, otherwise I get a seasick feeling. If they don't use the balls per guidelines, they lose the ball for their next turn. If there is a chronic problem, they lose it for a week. The balls sit on rubber rings at the end of the day so the custodian doesn't have to move balls to vacuum.*

My school, Crest View Elementary, has enough exercise balls in the gym that we can do practice games as a class where we pretend we are in the classroom and I am writing on the board. When I turn around, the students must be still with no big bounces on the ball. It's fun to make it into a game in physical education class and practice being still on the ball, so the students have time to work on their sitting position and posture on the ball as well as their ability to use small bounces or pulses, which are not a distraction to other students or the teacher. I have also promoted proper use of the balls by giving students a choice of active seating options when they are watching demonstrations, listening to instructions, or watching a short video clip in class. Integrating active seating into instruction teaches kids to advocate for their needs.

Once a teacher has two to six exercise balls in the classroom, I check in with the teacher and the students regularly to see how things are going. Sometimes we need to inflate or deflate the size of some of the balls to accommodate all the different students in terms of height and weight. Many times teachers end up adding more balls to the classroom as appropriate to accommodate their students.

DO I NEED A SPECIFIC GO-TO PERSON TO MANAGE THE EXERCISE BALLS?

We have learned from our experiences that the use of exercise balls needs to be coordinated, and both teachers and students need to feel comfortable. Having a go-to person to discuss and resolve any glitches that occur while integrating the balls into the classroom can simplify the process.

If you are a physical education teacher, specialist, administrator, or classroom teacher and you want to orchestrate the use of the balls in your school, you will need to keep the following things in mind:

- You will need a source of money to fund the program. (Details for gathering this funding appear in the next section in this chapter.)
- You will, of course, need the exercise balls themselves. (Information for ordering the exercise balls can be found in the appendix.)
- You will need an electric pump, plug pullers, and several Faster Blaster or dual-action hand pumps.

- Print the illustrations and guidelines for the correct sitting posture when using exercise balls that is provided on the CD-ROM in the back of this book. You may also use the illustrations and photos on the CD-ROM to create your own posters and overheads.
- Laminate the illustrations, photos, and guidelines, and have them ready for distribution.
- Be willing to put some time into getting the program started.
- Understand that the integration of the balls will take work. You will need to do the following:
    1. Order the exercise balls.
    2. Fill the balls with air.
    3. Train or give teachers reading materials, like this book, to help them get started.
    4. Distribute balls to those in the building who want to give the exercise balls a try in their rooms.
    5. Maintain the exercise balls, including occasionally organizing or making supplies available for ball cleaning. This is simple, and the students really like doing it. All you need is a nontoxic cleaner and some soft rags or cleaning cloths (see the appendix for a list of recommended cleaners). You can select a ball-cleaning crew, or make a station where kids can just go over and clean the balls as necessary.
- Finally, you need a desire to make a positive impact on your facility's learning environment. We think that's an admirable position to be in.

WHERE DO I FIND THE MONEY FOR EXERCISE BALLS, PUMPS, AND PLUG PULLERS?

Budgets can vary dramatically from one school or district to the next. Some educators may have access to an in-school grant process funded by a parent organization, and other educators will need to reach outside of their school for funding. Linda made good use of a public service grant in our area to purchase her exercise ball equipment. You may need to do a little research to find the money. We hope this book will be a good resource for showing your funding sources the rationale behind why you want to integrate the use of balls into your school. Meeting the growing needs of a diverse population and the research about positive connections between movement and learning are a strong place to start.

WHAT ARE THE REWARDS FOR USING EXERCISE BALLS IN THE CLASSROOM?

Some of the rewards for using exercise balls in the classroom are simply this: happy, focused, and productive kids. After reading through piles of student surveys (see more notes and quotes from kids later in this chapter), the overall consensus is that kids love choices and they love to move. In fact, research suggests children are hardwired to move (Healy 2004). As we discussed in part I of this book, sitting on the exercise balls increases blood circulation up and down the spinal column and to the brain. This increased circulation in turn oxygenates the blood the brain receives. Active sitting on the ball is great, and other active seating adaptations such as the discs, wedges, and cushions are also excellent choices. However and whatever you do to move more than you otherwise would is an improvement over being sedentary. The wedge specifically throws you a little forward so you are more upright, providing more space in the lungs for that oxygen you need to be more awake, alert, and productive. The disk offers that continual subtle movement in the hip area to maintain balance and stretch out the lower area of the back, which tends to tighten up when you sit still for a long time. Whether sitting on an exercise ball, disc, wedge, or cushion, movement increases focus and concentration. One of several studies I found on the Internet states the following: "For children with autism, therapy balls used for up to 10 minutes a day, for three weeks as an alternate form of classroom seating may improve in-seat behavior and attention to class activities by as little as 25% or as much as 80%" (Holman 2005).

When you implement the exercise ball program in such a way as to provide students with both the choices and the movement, then you have success. Not all kids think that exercise balls are "the best" and "totally rock" the way some do, and that is normal because we are all so different. The point is, the ones who do love them are pretty jazzed about the opportunity to sit on a ball in the classroom. Many kids and adults who have a great deal of trouble sitting still are given the chance on the ball to move in an appropriate way and get some exercise while situated in what many people and educators may have formerly seen as a sedentary environment. Some kids and adults whose "hard drives tend to go sleep" can be woken up and become more alert and awake after exercise that increases circulation (Jensen 1995). Time on the ball mimics other activities, such as taking a walk, by increasing circulation and bringing more oxygen to the brain.

Another reward for advocating for the use of exercise balls and active seating alternatives in schools and workplaces is a move towards a "motion promotion," which simply means integrating more movement throughout everyone's day. As Galen Cranz discusses at length in her book *The Chair* (2000), we need an environment that allows more movement throughout our day combined with intermittent rest as necessary to "recharge our batteries." We can't expect kids or adults to be sedentary most of the day and then go out after school or work and get enough physical activity to be their healthiest. We all need a variety of postures and movements throughout our day to feel our best.

Taking the stairs and parking the car farther away from your destination are good lifestyle choices to get us moving more. We want to encourage teachers to include even more movement opportunities throughout the day. Brain research recommends

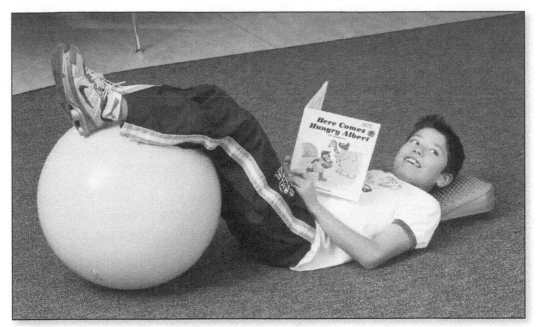

Aside from movement promotion in the classroom, the balls can also be used to rest and recharge our batteries.

that students and adults need to move approximately every 20 minutes (Jensen 2000). Movement improves brain development, increases nerve connections, and solidifies learning. Simple things like integrating more standing, stretching, and walking; having stools available; and having choices to sit, lie, or even crawl on the floor are important practices for teachers to incorporate into their teaching. Here's a list of some of our favorite quick-start activities to get the brain and body moving:

- **Integrate Brain Gym exercises into your day.** You can find more information from books listed in the appendix.

- **Surprise students with Movement Fire Drills throughout the day.** Choose an auditory signal, and instruct students that on the chosen signal, they should get up and look to you for a direction—wherein you point a finger right or left—and they do a quick lap around the room, finishing by sitting silently at their desks with hands flat on the desk in an X position.

- **Throw two- to three-minute dance parties.** You choose the song, put on the music, and everybody moves until the music stops. Choices can include kids choosing their own free-form movements or any of the following. The teacher leads these movements with actions and words while students "mimic" the specific move. (Idea from Katie Jones, first-grade teacher, personal communication):
  - *Arms in the air.*
  - *Let's go down low.*
  - *Let's jump up high.*
  - *Circle one way, then the other.*
  - Hand it over to the kids (when they have some moves) to come up and share.
  - You take it from here; let creativity reign.

- **Incorporate Volley Time into your day.** This is a "keep it up softly" activity. Have balloons or beach balls stashed in a closet or bag. When you're ready or in need of a movement break, bring out the objects of your choice—six or eight would be good—and place them on different desks. On your signal, the students stand and softly tap the objects to keep them up in the air and moving from student to student. Emphasize getting the object to everyone in the room. Once they have the game under control—including a stop signal—you can add music of your choice (adapted from Bevill 2003; Kim Bevill is a teacher, the founder of Gray Matters, and the creator of the Brain Basics Convention.)

Any activities involving quick movements are going to improve focus, learning, and productivity for everyone. It would be so beneficial for both classrooms and businesses to integrate more movement breaks into their day. What a fun and exciting way to improve student and staff morale!

ALTERNATIVE ACTIVE SEATING OPTIONS

As I mentioned earlier, I had an aha moment when I realized it really was a little crazy to ask teachers to start adding balls to their beautifully organized, well-run rooms. I'm talking about teachers who are masters and whom I admire and respect. So, when my friend and mentor Anne Turnacliff, who is retired and volunteers in my gym, gave a Hughes Basic Gross Motor Assessment to a student and recommended that the student start sitting on a wedge to build core strength, I thought *That's it.* This classroom teacher, a highly respected veteran, was fine with adding the wedge to this student's chair. I talked with the student and practiced with the wedge in the gym privately to be sure it was comfortable. Then the wedge was put in place in the classroom. When other students eventually asked about the wedge, the teacher told them it helped the student sit up straighter and focus, and the student smiled. That student is doing amazingly well. Other actions have been taken to help the student, and the combination of interventions has truly made a difference.

From that point, I started adding all the wedges and a disc I had to other classrooms. Cassie Zubiate-Rossi, a third-grade teacher who had balls in her room last year and again this year, is a member of our child assistance team (CAT) at Crest View Elementary. I have worked closely with her since last year when she added the balls as chairs to her room. Since that time, I have gone to CAT meetings in her room to discuss different students from different grade levels who were struggling with behaviors and academic problems in the gym and classroom settings.

Because Cassie is working to transition our school to the new RTIs (responses to interventions), we started meeting during our short and always interrupted lunch periods and laid out a plan to buy more wedges and discs and to add other sensory integration ideas. We knew we had to write a grant because our list was growing quickly. When I spoke with Amanda Betzen, our occupational therapist (OT) at Crestview Elementary, to fill her in on what Cassie and I were doing, she said, "We [Occupational Therapists] call those **sensory baskets.**" Amanda and I then brainstormed and wrote down ideas of things to add to the basket and how to get them for the best prices. Amanda is on a tight schedule, and I was ready to roll with the idea. I spent the weekend running around gathering stuff as inexpensively as I could to have at least two baskets ready by Monday. On Monday I brought the basket to Cassie, and she was excited and ready to start using some of the items in the basket right away. Now I needed to decide who else would want to field-test the second basket.

We have a first-grade teacher, Mandy Jasper, whom I had seen doing Brain Gym activities in her room and in the hallway with her students, and I thought, *Bingo*, she'd be a great teacher to share the second basket with. When I approached with the basket, she was happy. We went over what was in the basket and some ideas for how she could introduce the items, plus wedges and discs. She knew her students' needs very well, and she had some ideas of how she would start right away. I told her I'd need some feedback from her and the kids because we were writing a grant and wanted to get the baskets in more rooms as soon as possible. When I stopped back to see Mandy, our 1st grade teacher, later in the day, she was brimming over with good news, just as Cassie had been. Mandy had her first-grade students discussing the items in the basket, like little scientists. It couldn't have been more perfect. These sweet little kids were saying things like, "This wedge isn't really working that great for me. Can I trade you for the disc?" I knew that basket was well placed. The first week went on like that, and Amanda said that after a couple days the initial excitement had calmed to a productive hum. The items were being used, and Mandy—and her students—were more happy and productive.

The same scenario was happening in Cassie's room, with students coming into physical education commenting on how they loved the new items in the basket. Now I needed to actually buy more wedges and eventually discs to keep the ball rolling. I ordered a case of wedges on my VISA card and found homes for all 12 in different classrooms in no time. They were in 5th, 3rd, 2nd, and 1st grades. I already had balls in 4th grade and kindergarten. The motion promotion at Crest View Elementary was gaining momentum.

Following is a list of items that I included in the sensory baskets, which could actually be a crate, bag, backpack, or other similar item:

• **Sensory snakes:** A simple concept to weigh down the shoulders and neck area. They seem to calm people down. You can use tube socks for the cover and plastic newspaper bags as a liner for these. Fill the plastic newspaper bags with rice to make a weighted sock for the child to wear around their shoulders and neck. The weight or amount of rice should be light to medium (never too heavy—check with the child to be sure it feels o.k.) These sensory snakes or neck and shoulder weights can be decorated with snake eyes and a tongue. Years ago I worked with some PTs and OTs in Adams County District Number 12, and we made these to use with the kids. I'm not sure where the idea originated. I still like this idea because it's mostly recycled materials and made with inexpensive materials that you have on hand.

• **"Anne's Anchoring Ankrons"** (trademark and patent pending). I've been field-testing proto-types for my new "Anne's Anchoring Ankrons" shoulder and neck weights and lap pads for several months. I've also been changing the sizes and materials to customize them for specific age groups, desired outcomes, and activities. They are for people of all ages and can be placed around the shoulders and neck and the lap. Field testing results on folks of all ages have found that they seem to relax, ground, and keep folks in their seat and productive a little longer.

• "Anne's Anchoring Ankrons" are meant to be used intermittently during the day and evening. According to Amanda Betzen, our OT, these weighted type objects should never weigh more than 25% of a person's total body weight. The bottom line is the teachers and the kids that I've been testing them with seem to love them. My principal, Ned Levine, jokingly said he'd like 600 of them because they seem to calm all of us down—both teachers and kids.

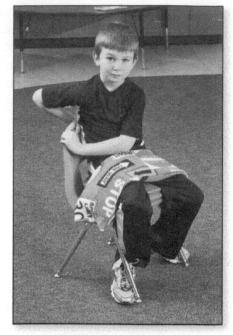

• **Aromatherapy calming or exciting smells**: Students self-select the smells according to what's appealing to them. To provide these smells, use a variety of essential oils, cotton balls, and sandwich bags or plastic film containers to keep them fresh. Do a scientific "sniff-off," and have students choose the smell they like best. Add a few drops of the oil, and place the cotton ball in the sandwich bag or film container. Children may keep the aromatherapy packets or film containers in their desks and use them as necessary as long as they're not a distractor factor.

• **Chewlery**: Chewlery is a patented jewelry collection that includes necklaces, pins, and bracelets that can be safely chewed to relieve stress or motor or oral overflow.

• **Chopsticks and large jacks**: Students use the chopsticks to pick up the large jacks and place them in other containers. These are great for coordination and agility using the hands and for fine motor skills. They're also great when you need another novel idea for a math manipulative.

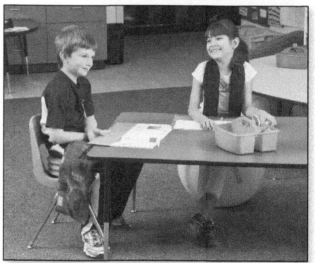

Anne's Anchoring Ankrons lap pad and Anne's Anchoring Ankrons neck weight in use.

• **Blindfolds and bags of different items**: Students can reach in and touch to feel an item and then guess what they think it is. Items can be changed to address any appropriate subject being taught. For example, nutrition teachers could use fruits and vegetables; geometry teachers could use shapes; and science teachers could promote kinesthetic awareness with items that are smooth, rough, soft, cuddly, and so on.

• **Discs and wedges**: These will increase balance, strength, focus, and state of alertness as well as improve posture and proprioception. Proprioception is like a GPS system for the body. There are sensors located in the muscles, tendons, joints, and inner ear that allow us to know where we are in space.

•**Air cushions**: These options for active seating add movement and comfort to the classroom.

•**Putty and modeling clay**: Putty and modeling clay relieve anxiety and stress while strengthening hands.

As you can guess, the list could go on forever. Think about stimulating the senses, and keep adding to your baskets as you discover items that fit your needs and those of your students.

HOW DO KIDS FEEL ABOUT USING EXERCISE BALLS IN THEIR CLASSES?

As previously mentioned, we had seven different classrooms using the exercise balls in my school last year. I was able to summarize student comments from all grade levels; the following list covers comments from kindergarten through fifth grade. I asked each student, "What do you like about having the balls in your classroom?" Here are some of their responses:

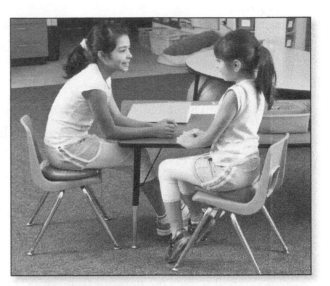

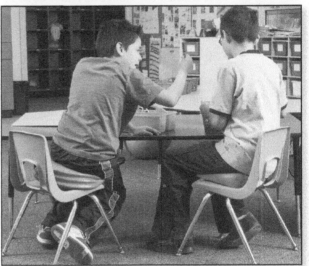

Disc, air cushion, and wedges in use.

- "We have a break from reagler [regular] chairs."
- "I think they help your body."
- "I like it because it helps me constetrax [concentrate]."
- "I like it because they are fun and good for muscular strength and endurance."
- "They are comferting [comforting]."
- "It gives me something different to sit on."
- "I relax better on a ball than a chair."
- "I like that you can bounce a little."
- "Fun to sit on."
- "It's fun to bounce 'smally' when the teacher is writing on the board."
- "They are fun and they make me happy."
- "I like trying to have a straight back."
- "I like that they are rubbery and cool to sit on."

- "I like them because they use the muscles in your back a lot."
- "Me gusta tener las pelotas porque hago ejercisio." (I like the ball because I can exercise.)
- "The ball helps me focus."
- "I like the balls because they are good for balance and control."
- "I like to have the ball because you have to use lots of your musels [muscles]."
- "I like that they give us a challenge."
- "I like it because I pay more attention to my teacher."

There are a few kids who do not like using the ball, and their comments are as follows:

- "It's too much bouncing."
- "It makes me nervous that I could tip." (*Note:* Exercise balls are not for everyone, and if teachers have a rotation system, students are free to pass and not take a turn.)
- "It doesn't feel good to my back."
- "I don't like when they roll out from under me." (*Note:* We're primarily using balls with feet now, and the rolling problem has been solved.)
- "Sometimes they are a distraction and annoying." (*Note:* We're working on being more proactive with this one. This needs to be addressed quickly if it happens.)
- "I don't like how rarely I get a turn." (*Note:* We feel your pain and are working to have more balls available on request.)

HOW DO TEACHERS FEEL ABOUT USING EXERCISE BALLS IN THEIR CLASSES?

The specific question I asked teachers was, "How have the balls affected your classroom?"

- "I think they help the kids concentrate more. The kids love them, and adults in the room comment on how they'd never know balls were there if I did not point it out."—Renee Cerny, kindergarten
- "It has added a whole new dimension to learning—a positive choice. They make the room more fun/friendly."—Jeri Eurich, SIED teacher
- "It seems to help more active kids relax . . . but not all of them."—Cindy Monnet, fourth grade
- "The kids seem to stay very alert 'on the ball'—no slouching. Also it's an interesting 'comfy' option for different styles of kids."—Erin Shea Bower, fifth grade
- "Many kids use the balls properly and enjoy sitting on them. They are eager for their day. They do not cause a significant behavior problem as the class knows if they misuse the ball, they lose it for the day."—Peter Mitchell, first grade

Adding exercise balls to your classroom takes a concerted effort. It also takes organization and management. For many children, it does help them focus and concentrate, and as the kids said repeatedly in their surveys, it gives them a choice, a chance to move more, and a break from traditional hard chairs.

Finally, here are two teachers' responses to the question "Would you recommend other teachers try having this alternative seating option available in their rooms?" Both said yes, and their comments follow:

• "Yes, the balls work great if the teacher's attitude and style fits this idea. My biggest concern initially was how to manage it without too much disruption to others in the class. After a couple short lessons, that turned out to be a nonissue. If someone is not using the ball correctly I just say, 'Time to pass the ball,' and the problem is over. Once we set up a procedure, it went well. The small laminated visual is also passed to the next student on the ball, so students can be constantly aware of proper sitting and behavior in the class. I can't imagine my class without balls now!" —Donna Casey, fourth grade. (*Note:* The illustration of how to sit on the ball correctly is available on the bound-in CD-ROM.)

• "No matter how you decide to implement these, there are kids who can use them properly and derive a benefit." —Peter Mitchell, first grade

Responses to the wedges, discs, and air cushions have been favorable from a variety of kids and teachers in my school. This is excellent news on the motion promotion front because there are no more hesitations about active seating.

SUMMARY

Integrating exercise balls, alternative active seating options, and sensory baskets in the classroom could involve a go-to person, money, time, energy, and strategizing. You could also do it alone to get things started more quickly. It's really not that difficult, expensive, or time consuming. And later if you want to go schoolwide, you'll be ready. Either way, we think it is well worth the effort!

We've saved the best for last, so you can read it now or save it for later, but do read the final chapter. Chapter 14, "Balancing Our Lives at Home and at Work Using Active Seating and Sensory Baskets," is sure to shed some light on regulating your way through the day.

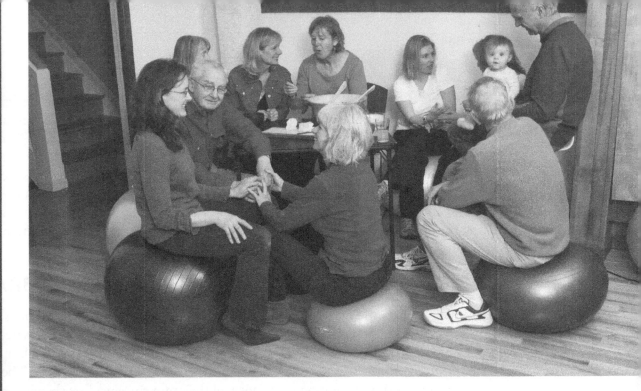

fourteen

Balancing Our Lives at Home and at Work Using Active Seating and Sensory Baskets

*H*ope is a waking dream. —*Aristotle*

Many of us have been talking about time management and balancing our lives for a long time. In the January edition of *O, the Oprah Magazine* in the "What I Know for Sure" section, Oprah states the following (Winfrey 2009): "Everything I know for sure about maintaining a sense of balance and well-being, I allowed to be pushed aside to make room for whatever was masquerading as a priority. I took myself off my to-do list; whatever time was left over is what I gave myself." Oprah refers to this imbalance in her life as "falling off the wagon." We hear you, Oprah; at times we've even felt as if our wagon wheels have fallen off.

Multitasking and juggling events sometimes leaves us feeling exhausted, unfulfilled, and even disconnected from our loved ones. Anxiety, fear of change, and lack of time can be overriding factors in transforming our lives from poor emotional and physical health to living well.

Incorporating simple strategies and tools to achieve a more active lifestyle may be easier than you think. Changing your stationary seating to disks and wedges is inexpensive and can be quickly adapted to your home and work environment. Customizing a sensory basket will give you more energy to complete daily activities. Bouncing and stretching on your exercise ball intermittently throughout your ordinarily sedentary moments can be refreshing. Why not incorporate a ball for your children to sit on at the computer desk, place a disk in the seat of your grandmother's wheelchair, or ask the boss if exercise balls could be available in the office break room? These steps can be life changing.

EMOTIONS, PHYSICAL ACTIVITY, AND YOUR BRAIN

Human beings are amazingly adaptable. In the book *The Brain That Changes Itself*, Norman Doidge, MD, speaks to the issue of how the brain can "change, rewire, rearrange, and grow" (Doidge 2007, p. xx). Doidge states, "The idea that the brain can change in its own structure and function through thought and activity is, I believe, the most important alteration in our view of the brain since we first sketched out its basic anatomy and the workings of its basic component, the neuron" (pp. xv and xvi). Doidge continues to emphasize that "the neuroplastic revolution has implications for, among other things, our understanding of how love, sex, grief, relationships, learning, addictions, culture, technology, and psychotherapies change our brains" (pp. xvi). Doidge also makes the connection between physical exercise and learning, saying, "Thus physical exercise and learning work in complementary ways: the first to make new stem cells, the second to prolong their survival" (pp. 252-253).

The interconnectedness of our brains with thoughts, emotions, and movement affecting us in ongoing and continuous manners is being proven repeatedly in different settings. From the office and home environment all the way to prisons and correctional facilities, every person is capable of change. Awakening to the concept that our bodies, brains, and emotions are not permanently hardwired is hopeful. And that is why I'm going to share two book talks that occurred within a one-week period, both of which connected the critical emotional states of mind with crisis and the optimism of these two authors.

Nationally honored teacher and best-selling author Wally Lamb was the first of the two authors I (Anne) was lucky enough to hear, Marc Bekoff was the second to speak at the Boulder Bookstore in December 2008. The book Wally was speaking about was *The Hour I First Believed*. In the book, a school nurse survives the Columbine High School massacre. In his talk at the store, Lamb discussed crisis situations in our society and how emotional breakdowns affect our society. He discussed another one of his books, *Couldn't Keep It to Myself*, in which he shares a collection of stories written by his students at York Correctional Institute. The female prisoners of York describe "how they were imprisoned by abuse, rejection, and their own self-destructive impulses long before they entered the criminal justice system" (Lamb 2004). When he facilitates the expression of thoughts and emotions with the women through their writing, it allows them to have a voice and to feel the potential for change. Paying attention to people's emotional state is critical. These facilities have exercise areas, which acknowledge the prisoners' need to move and play as human beings. Now the question is this: Could we integrate more movement into their days in these correctional facilities? Is the cost reasonable, and could it help their rehabilitation process?

Within a week of Wally Lamb's appearance, one of the world's foremost experts on animal emotions, Marc Bekoff, was discussing his children's book *Animals at Play: Rules of the Game*. In this book, Bekoff states, "Why do young animals play? Their play is for exercise, gaining strength, and developing muscles for when they grow older, so they can run long distances and run fast. . . . Playing is also a time for learning" (Bekoff 2008, p. 6).

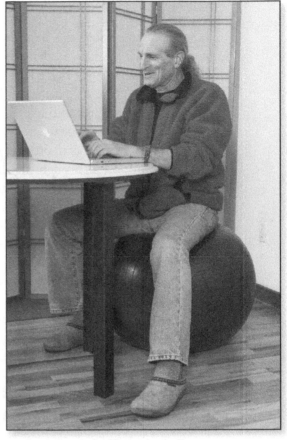

Doidge also reinforces this need for exercise in animals: "We now know that exercise and mental activity in animals generate and sustain more brain cells, and we have many studies confirming that humans that lead mentally active lives have better brain functioning" (Doidge 2007, p. 254).

Bekoff, like Wally Lamb, works in a program that reaches out to a correctional facility. In Marc's case, he is working at the Boulder County Jail with Jane Goodall's Roots & Shoots program. He is a roving ambassador. At the jail, he teaches animal behavior, conservation biology, and animal and environmental ethics to a group of male prisoners. In the program, the men he works with write letters and poems telling kids about the mistakes they've made and how jail is not the best place to make a difference in the world. In *Animals at Play: Rules of the Game*, Bekoff emphasizes fair play and the significance of cooperation and

Author Marc Bekoff, on the ball.

justice. The audience questions at Marc's book talk turned, as they did at Wally's, to the topics of crisis, control, our schools, and our children:

- Are we taking away recess when kids need the exercise and the time to play more than ever?
- Do they need play time to learn about social behaviors they'll need throughout life?
- Are kids being allowed to goof off and have fun, or are they being placed on athletic teams and organized activities too early in life?
- Are our kids getting time when they are not in school to play in the neighborhood?
- Are there any kids in the neighborhood to play with if your child is home, or is everyone else in those organized activities?

- Do kids know the rules of the game and know how to play fair?
- Are individuals at home and work playing fair? Do they know the rules? Are they getting enough exercise? Are you integrating play and exercise into your day?

My connecting point to all this is that acting upon knowledge, information, and an understanding of our physical and emotional potential can teach us to manage our time, our bodies, and our emotions. This includes daily fluctuations in energy, mood, and emotion. Regulating our way through the day with the help of active seating and sensory baskets is a step toward self-control, something that is often talked about but not always fully understood. Unfortunately, some people end up regulating their systems with risky behavior and sometimes substance abuse. When physical and psychological needs are met with healthy choices, the possibilities and creative avenues for a productive and happy life are endless.

Our bodies and the way we treat them are like our friendships or bank accounts. We have to make deposits in order to make withdrawals. If we take care of our bodies and exercise our way through the day, they will be strong. When or if something goes wrong, we'll hopefully be strong enough to fight it. If we munch our way healthfully through the day making careful choices about what we eat, we may weigh less, have more energy, and feel better. Friends need healthy deposits, acts of kindness, birthday celebrations, invitations to do fun things, and a thank-you note or e-mail taking notice of the things we like about them on occasion. We don't make friendship deposits so we can make withdrawals later, but it does kind of work that way. If we haven't made enough deposits and our friends don't feel loved and supported, they're not as inclined to come running when we need them. If we spend more money than we have in our bank accounts we'll go into debt, and that won't feel good either. The idea of making deposits rather than withdrawals is very powerful and empowering.

TRUE STORY TIME: SOMEWHAT UNHEALTHY WAYS OF REGULATING OUR WAY THROUGH PAIN

When I blew out my ankle several years ago, I was in some serious chronic pain for a really long time. Over the course of about two years, my ankle was casted and booted intermittently, and I was not getting my usual dose of exercise and the natural release of those feel-good hormones we get when we move enough. I had many mindless moments of munching that led me to gain weight like I never had before. The weight slowed me down, and combined with the pain and lack of movement, I was experiencing something I never understood before. I understood what depression was. My moods plummeted, and I experienced more moments of mindless munching and more weight gain.

Martha Spaulding, my physical therapist at the time, was wonderful, empathetic, kind, and knowledgeable. One day I mentioned that my weight gain was killing me, and she made a very wise and true statement. She said, "You know, if you wore some pants that you could actually feel on your body . . ." What I inferred from that was "Stop wearing the sweatpants you've been living in since you injured your ankle." The pants were so comfortable that I felt comfortable eating in them nonstop. I think this involved sensory integration because when I could feel my body in my new pants, it was a signal to stop eating when they got a little snug. I needed to stop eating to try to feel good because the extra food didn't really make me feel better. The eating made me feel worse because it was not making the pain go away or making it easier to move on crutches.

I lost 40 pounds, and I am happy and active again, but I'll never forget what it felt like to be depressed and over a comfortable weight for me. I was making deposits of food and added calories without the withdrawals I used to make when I was moving all the time. Our weight is related to a combination of genetics and how much and what we eat, as well as how much, how often, and how hard we exercise or move. If we increase our movement and make healthy choices about how much and what we eat, we'll feel better. The feeling better is much more important than the number on the scale. Often, the simplest movement activities such as bouncing on an exercise ball or sitting on a wedge can improve our well-being.

AN IMPORTANT POINT ON WEIGHT AND EXERCISE: DO WE HAVE TO BE FIT TO FIT IN?

As a physical educator, I have never been terribly fond of fitness tests that say if you can't do this number of push-ups or pull-ups, or run a mile in this amount of time, you're out of shape, and you have to do more and do it harder to get in shape. The out-of-shape people give up, thinking, *The hill is too steep and I'm not going to make it, so I'll just sit down and give up.* I've seen it repeatedly in people of all ages, and I believe it is at least part of the reason for the obesity crisis we have right now in America. We scare people. We say, "Go faster and harder, more, more, that's not good enough," and people slowly inch back to the couch or chair and remain sedentary.

Sadly, at times, I've been in fitness facilities and classes where it felt as if the instructor wasn't always tuning in to the needs of all the students. People who are self-conscious about their weight in the first place need personal attention and more encouragement than some of the people in the fitness classes and health clubs who are super fit. People of all sizes and shapes should be encouraged and paid attention to, so they don't just poof and disappear back into their sedentary lives because it didn't feel as if they were making progress or losing weight. Personal trainers are a great idea and a good investment. Some clubs are now offering time with personal trainers for reduced rates, or they include an initial consultation to get you started. This individualized time is critical to success. It helps people really tune in to their bodies and the areas they need to work on, like core strength, which the exercise ball does such a great job of strengthening in such a variety of fun ways. In Boulder, I see recreation centers and health clubs that use exercise balls and include ball classes as part of their exercise programs.

GREAT REASONS THE BALLS WORK FOR ALL AGES

People who want to be social can attend those exercise ball classes we just mentioned. Check your area for exercise ball classes available at recreation centers and clubs. Others who want to stay home can use the exercises found in part II of this book and the photos and illustrations on the CD-ROM in the back of this book to pick out exercises to focus on for a week, or however long it feels right, then change it up with choices from the different categories found in chapters 5 through 10.

Another suggestion for at-home users is a great instructional video called *FitBall: The Balanced Workout*. I've used this program at home and with students of different ages, and it's always a big hit. There are three different people demonstrating, a man and two women, and they show each exercise with correct form and at three different levels of performance including beginning, intermediate, and advanced. (See the resources for a description and ordering information for this video or DVD.) Lindsay Zappala and Joanne Posner-Mayer, physical therapist and our coauthor from *Kids on the Ball* (Spalding et al. 1999), designed the instructional video. They did an impressive job with the design and production of this video, and it's a total-body workout using the exercise ball that has stood the test of time; as other DVDs have been produced, *FitBall: The Balanced Workout* is still holding its own because it's well done. Lindsay is one of the owners of Body Dynamics, a studio in Boulder where she teaches exercise ball classes, Pilates mat classes, and my favorite, Pilates on the reformer. Lindsay is one teacher whom I have stuck with for the last 20-some years because she does pay attention to every student in every class. She makes sure that everyone's form is correct. She zeros in on what you need as a person with unique needs. I would highly recommend that trainers and individuals make it a point to come take a class or observe her in action because she puts theory into practice, with the biomechanics of exercise up front and center.

Exercise balls offer a place for active sitting. They can help us calm down or maintain an alert state, all while improving core strength. The opportunity to improve our overall fitness level and our sense of balance throughout our day at work and at home is a good reason to have this inexpensive item as part of our work and home environments.

Galen Cranz, PhD, professor of architecture at the University of California at Berkeley, wrote a book called *The Chair: Rethinking Culture, Body, and Design*. In the book, Dr. Cranz does an incredible job of researching and discussing chairs, historically and culturally, and how they affect our bodies and our minds at home, work, and school. Her book reinforces our thoughts and feelings in relation to personal fitness and everyday life. In the final chapter of her book, Dr. Cranz discusses changing lifestyles and describes her ideal workplace. In the description, she mentions using a ball: "The thing in the office that might make you most curious is related to exercise: a large inflated ball over which staff members occasionally drape themselves to promote flexibility of the spine. Some sit on it in lieu of a stool" (Cranz 2000, p. 220).

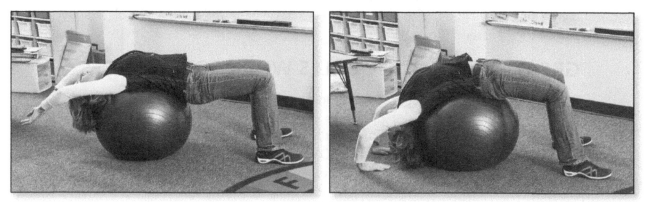

Tracy Halgren, parent and active community volunteer, takes a stretch break on the ball.

USING EXERCISE BALLS THROUGH THE PHASES OF LIFE: BIRTH, MIDLIFE, LATER IN LIFE

People of all ages are "hardwired" to move. We move to meet our basic needs, to increase alertness, to explore our surroundings, to improve our fitness, and so on. Using exercise balls through different phases of our lives helps us to regulate our way through the day and our need to move.

Using Exercise Balls for Newborns

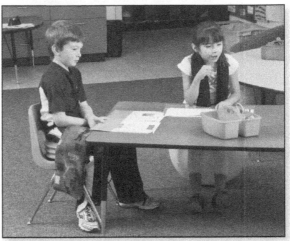

We're born and we're dependent; we need assistance to find food (a mother's guiding hand to her breast) and to find comfort when something hurts (from Mom or Dad). The hardest thing for parents and other family members is when the new baby is crying, and no one can figure out why. They try everything to no avail. Everyone is sleep deprived. They're calling friends, reading books, and finally going to the doctor when nothing else works.

Active seating for all ages.

One of my fourth-grade students, Bergen, mentioned that they had "one of those big balls" in their house but it was just for mom, dad, and their new baby. The baby, Fielden, was clearly a bright light in Bergen's life, and I wanted to know more about the ball and it's connection to the family. I called Bergen's mother, Melissa, and she was more than happy to fill me in. Fielden was born with esophagitis—what many of us know as acid reflux. It makes it hard for him to sleep through the night. He was crying from 2:00 a.m. to 5:00 a.m. or from 3:00 a.m. to 6:00 a.m., and he was inconsolable. Fielden was a cranky baby because he was in pain. That was extremely difficult on Mom and the whole family.

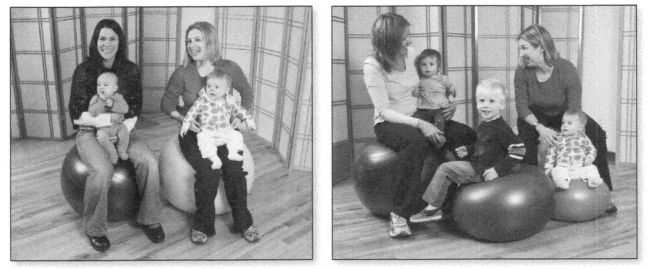

Using an exercise ball with your infant or young child makes for happy babies and moms!

While we were writing *Kids on the Ball: Using Swiss Balls in a Complete Fitness Program*, our coauthor and physical therapist friend Joanne Posner-Mayer gave each of us a small, thin book by Sheila M. Frick (1996) called *Out of the Mouths of Babes: Discovering the Developmental Significance of the Mouth—A Book Especially for Parents & Other "Grown-Ups."* This book has been enormously helpful in explaining in easy-to-understand language what was happening with my student Bergen's family and their baby, Fielden. In the book, we all learned something that would stick with us forever. An acronym, SSB, or "suck/swallow/breathe (SSB) synchrony" (Frick 1996, p. 4) that we would find rolling off our tongues because it makes so much sense. I'll put it in my own words here: When we're trying to organize ourselves and focus, we need air. To get more air, we suck in the air in whatever manner works for us at the moment. Next, we have to swallow and exhale. The synchrony part is like integration, pulling it all together in a smooth move. The problem is that it's not always easy to make it a smooth move, and some of us need more intense energy to focus in the first place. When things get hard, like when Fielden was experiencing reflux, he needed some outside help to regulate or synchronize his suck, swallow, and breathe. The SSB mechanism was not naturally kicking in because it hurt to suck, swallow, and try to breathe.

When his mom, Melissa, took him to the doctor, they were sent to a speech pathologist at the Mapleton Rehabilitation center here in Boulder. Speech pathologist Alison Stamn got things rolling quickly. She told Melissa she needed to get an exercise ball as soon as possible, and she did. Alison explained that the bouncing motion when sitting on the exercise ball holding the baby provides a soothing rhythm to help Fielden regulate his SSB and help him get past the reflux. The gentle bouncing motion would also soothe him and help him get back to sleep. Melissa said that when she held Fielden while she bounced, pushing gently from her feet, he responded immediately. They also use the ball to bounce the baby at dinner time. It's hard to imagine that a gentle bounce on the ball could help regulate breathing and calm a fussy baby who isn't reponding to rocking and other strategies. It's that up and down rhythm that is easily created when sitting on the ball that does it.

Alison the speech pathologist shared with Melissa that she gets all her friends who have babies an exercise ball for a baby shower gift. The gift is priceless when that little bundle of joy is finally sleeping in your arms. We think Alison is correct, and we'll be giving exercise balls to those new moms we know from now on.

In *Out of the Mouths of Babes*, Frick follows the SSB synchrony throughout life and shows how as we age, we just shift the items we put in our mouths to help us focus. Think about if you've ever been around kids who suck on their shirt sleeves, collars, or necklaces. As teachers we see it all the time. It's not a bad thing. It's just a sign that a child may be having to work extra hard to complete whatever task it is he is working on. For all of us, some things are easy and other things a challenge. When I played competitive basketball, I vividly remember having my tongue out as I dribbled downcourt, trying to get and keep my focus. I was also a nail-biter, a habit I've gotten over.

Now back to kids and helping them find their focus in relation to the active seating options and sensory baskets. You can look back at chapter 13 to see the suggestions we make for time at school. In the following section, you'll find more information on to how to make a few additions to your home to make it an even more fun place for kids to play.

Using Exercise Balls for Children

Very young children learn about balance by exploring their environments and can have a wonderful time with the addition of large balls and active seating devices, like the donuts in the photo, in the home as an interactive piece of exercise equipment or as an additional choice for seating, in lieu of a stool or chair. It is important to have the proper size ball for younger children and to use the ball on a carpeted or padded surface. See chapter 2 for recommendations on getting a ball that fits. An adult can assist a child with safe exploration and interactive activities on the exercise ball. On the CD-ROM in the back of this book, you will find all of our exercises and ideas from the first book, *Kids on the Ball* (Spalding et al. 1999).

Sensory Baskets: Helping You and Your Family Regulate Your Way Through the Day

Let's start with the kids and something that's really important for helping them regulate their way through the day. Having friends and being a friend is very important to a child. Play dates are not easy for all kids. Everyone is different, and it's good to know and recognize the needs of your own kids and their friends. That way you can set your children up to suceed when they get invited to play in different locations. Knowing what keeps your children happy and in their best state of mind allows you to send a few items along on play dates that can help them feel comfortable when away from home. Hopefully the play dates will run smoothly, because play and friends are essential to life. The degrees of friendship and the frequency of visits will vary depending on the child. People and kids with autism, Asperger's, and other extra challenges will need to be coached a little more. Parents can find books on these topics by doing searches on the computer or talking to a school therapist. Professional guidance is necessary to be sure we're not pushing at the wrong time or in the wrong way when working with kids with special needs.

Sensory baskets are also something that may come in handy when you are around other families that could use a little help regulating their way through the day. It's always touchy to give others advice, and none of us wants to come off as a know-it-all. I try to use the approach I take in class with the kids, asking if I can suggest something I saw work for someone else. It's good to give people choices because sometimes we're just not wanting any advice. Other times, when the timing is just right, we're so relieved for an idea to make a chaotic day a little calmer that we jump on a suggestion from a friend or friendly onlooker (that's what a lot of us who are teachers and who do or don't have kids consider ourselves, especially when we're bursting to give one little tidbit of information that might help).

The Concept of a Sensory Basket in the Home and on the Road

Parents usually already have bags they take places with their babies and toddlers. The bags usually have things like crunchy snacks; water, milk, or juice; and often a set of clean clothes for those wet, cold, or messy times that some of us love. A sensory basket is a basket, bag, backpack, crate, or other carrying device that you put specific things in that help you and the kids regulate your way through the day. Integrating your senses is really about reflecting on what you smell, feel, hear, touch, taste, and see that calms or excites you as you see the need. It helps you feel happy and allows you and the kids to enjoy yourselves wherever you go. The items that follow can be found at home or ready to go on the road. Everyone's sensory basket can include items that are customized to the senses by selecting things each person likes from the different categories.

- Tasting
    - Healthy vegetables or fruit
    - Healthy crunchy things such as popcorn or crackers
    - Water
    - Juice or milk
- Smelling
    - Aromatherapy (see chapter 13 for cotton ball ideas)
    - A favorite lotion with a calming or exciting scent
    - Lemons or oranges for the natural scent, and you can eat or use them later
- Seeing
    - Books
    - Puzzles
    - Fun flash cards
- Feeling
    - Favorite stuffed animal
    - Blanket
    - Squeaky toy (turn off the sound effects if you don't want to disturb the driver in the car)
    - Balls that are fun to fidget with; they sometimes have strings or nubs and can be soft, medium, or firm
    - Putty (the kind that doesn't stick to everything)
    - Lap pad (see description on page 211 in chapter 13)
    - Sensory snake (see description on page 211 in chapter 13)
- Hearing
    - MP3, disc, or tape player with headphones
    - Favorite music
    - Books on disc or MP3 player
    - Earplugs or sound-eliminating headphones for needed quite time

Using Exercise Balls as Adults in the Workplace

We spoke in an earlier chapter about being sensitive to those around you if you're going to add a ball to your work space. If you think it might intrude on other people's space or be a distractor factor, you should talk to those involved. Use common sense and be sensitive. You can even put sticky notes on the pages of this book and let others read about it for themselves. And a picture is always worth a thousand words, so do show the pictures in figure 14.1 so they know it's not really that "out there."

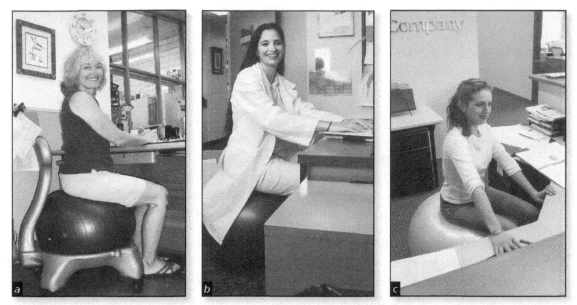

Figure 14.1 People we caught "on the ball" during their workday: *(a)* Bev Buchler, principal's secretary; *(b)* Angie Jouaneh, PA-C, dermatology; *(c)* Nicole Reno, branch facilitator of a mortgage company.

© Anne Spalding

Using Exercise Balls in Midlife: Sensory Parties

Let's talk about adults and something that's really important to them—fostering relationships through playful, fun activities. As the years go by, many adults enjoy different kinds of get-togethers and parties to suit their needs and interests. Some want to include traditional movement, dancing, and of course music, but we suggest expanding the party themes to deliberately include more of our senses. How about a sensory party?

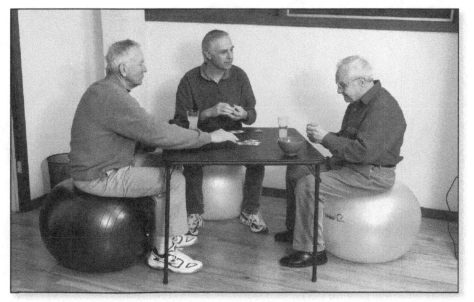

Boys playing cards on the ball.

What would a sensory party look like? There are lots of variations. I've hosted a few of these, and they've been very memorable. So, read the list, and see if any of these look like something you might want to include in a party with your friends. Keep in mind with these party suggestions that active seating is interesting and fun and makes a great addition to any of the following gatherings.

•**Active seating party**. If you already have some of these active seating options, make them available to your friends, and we know it will be a conversation starter. If it's a gift-giving occasion, maybe you'll give the guest of honor a disk, a wedge, a cushion, or an exercise ball. The CD-ROM in the back of this book includes our games and dance chapter activities from our book *Kids on the Ball* that can be easily incorporated to liven up the party.

•**Kick back and soak your feet**. That's right, we all got together and brought tubs and buckets or those vibrating tubs that warm the water like a real pedicure. We soaked our feet and used the tools they would use at a place that gives pedicures, but we just hung out and did it at my house. Those who were into color took turns painting each other's toes. We talked, laughed, ate some healthy snacks, and had a great afternoon hanging out and tuning in to each other and our feet.

•**Chair or table massages**. Boulder has a great massage school, and we have lots of people licensed to give massages, along with students who need to get in their hours working on people to get through the massage programs. Either way, having a masseuse or masseur come to your house might not be as expensive as you think. Everyone kicks in for their 30 minutes or so, and everyone leaves relaxed and happy.

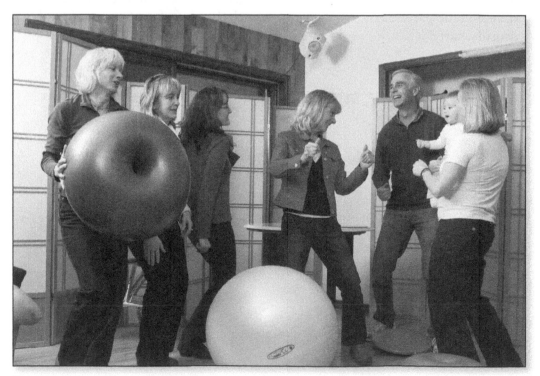

Dancing at an active seating party.

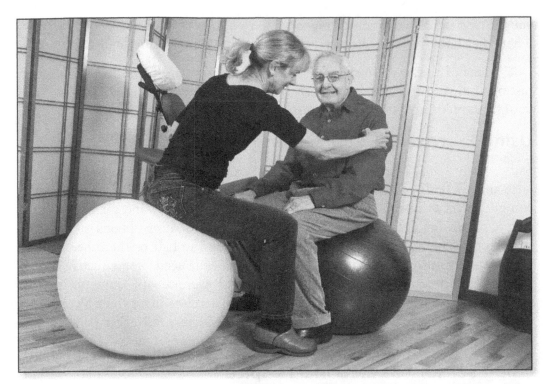

In home massage therapy on the ball.

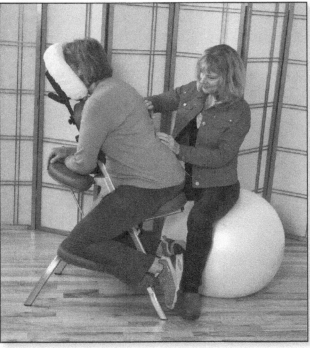

•**Tamale making**. Our friend Theresa is from Mexico, and she invited some friends over one Christmas to learn how to make homemade tamales. It was quite a sensory experience as we took turns with our hands in the *masa* (dough) made of cornmeal that we spread and wrapped around the filling. The tasting part was heaven. We recently had a repeat of that party; this time we went vegetarian with our fillings, and they were great.

•**Sensory birthday party**. Everyone brings an item to put in a sensory basket for the birthday person. The gifts don't have to fit in the basket. Like the shower gift for new moms, an exercise ball makes a great sensory gift. A wedge, disk, or air cushion to promote active sitting are more winning ideas that make healthy gifts. Aromatherapy lamps and environmentally friendly candles would also be good choices.

•**Soup party**. I'm planning a soup party, and I can smell it now. I want to combine it with those wonderful chair massages. We can all stay in the same room if people want to hear the conversation during the massages. They do it at Whole Foods Market, where they have the little cafe where people are eating and talking. Why not at home?

The idea of all these events is to focus on the senses: smelling, touching, feeling, tasting, and seeing. The sensory parties are always unique because you customize your focus on things you think will bring joy to your senses and your friends' senses.

Using Exercise Balls for Seniors

Sadly, many seniors survive things such as bypass surgery only to lose their balance and fall and break a hip or other bone. These accidents can sometimes lead to complications and death. This is a devastating circumstance, and we want to be a part of promoting the use of the exercise ball and active seating options in our aging population. The added movement gained by using the ball or the other options intermittently during the day will help accommodate the need for more active sitting, postural adjustments, and a sense of balance. The exercise ball, donut, or peanut are also suitable for strengthening and stretching exercises that can be a part of an everyday commitment to fitness. See chapters 6 and 10, respectively, in part II of this book for exercises. Safety and comfort are particularly important for seniors.

Using Sensory Baskets in a Hospice

My friend Jane Glassman Cohen, a transformational therapist extraordinaire, works for HospiceCare of Boulder and Broomfield Counties in Boulder, Colorado. When I was telling Jane about the sensory baskets I was making for the classrooms at my school, she shared with me how they use sensory baskets in the hospice program here in Boulder.

They have baskets with themes, such as the beach, the farm, and the kitchen. Each basket has things that people can smell, feel, hear, see, and sometimes taste that fit the theme. This is an incredible way to help people who are dying, and sometimes in pain, to feel a little calmer and hopefully a little happier during their final days on earth, including people experiencing memory loss or Alzheimer's, people with various stages of dementia, or people who are challenging to communicate with in ordinary ways.

People who are dying can still smile while holding something soft, warm, or familiar. Items such as pinecones or rocks seemed unusual to me at first. Then I thought more about our baskets for the students, and how much fun they might have closing their eyes or wearing a blindfold and guessing what items were in the container. The rocks or pinecones could be used when studying earth science. The sensory baskets bring back memories through the senses: the smell of evergreen, the feel of sand, or the sound of a favorite old song. Connecting the young and old and how the same things make sense and hold meaning for us brought more light to this concept.

The list of simple, easy-to-gather items is endless. The fact that these items can bring pleasure and trigger happy memories in the brain brings hope of a less scary experience when the inevitable end of our lives comes. All I could say as Jane explained the use of the baskets was, "I want a sensory basket by my side when I'm saying good-bye." What a lovely idea. It's not that expensive or difficult to put together, and the happiness it brings is so pure and simple—absolutely perfect.

Another aspect of the sensory assistance that HospiceCare brings to the Boulder area occurs at the Care Center, an inpatient unit for people who are actively dying or who have pain or other symptoms out of control and need 24-hour care. One of the things I think is brilliant about the program is the aromatherapy aspect. Jane told me they use Crock-Pots with water and essential oils to hold warm towels. Patients have the opportunity to use these warm, scented towels as part of their Comfort Care inpatient program. This gives the patients a chance to breathe in different moist and delicious smells, such as lavender, rosemary, peppermint, or cinnamon, as they use the towels at different times during the day. You can find more information about HospiceCare of Boulder and Broomfield Counties in Boulder, Colorado, at http://hospicecareonline.org.

Final Thoughts on Using Exercises Balls in All Phases of Life

The preceding sensory suggestions and ideas can be mixed and used to make you feel good now. What a concept, taking care of ourselves right now because it's the right thing to do. If we don't take care of ourselves and treat ourselves with kindness, we can't be there for our loved ones. So, here's to self-care—don't wait. Start adding more things that you like to see, smell, hear, and feel to your daily life. Shake it up, mix it up, and share ideas with your friends. Start with an active seating option, and add items to your personalized sensory basket, so you can regulate your way through the day. Hopefully, your days will get more relaxed, fun, and productive.

SUMMARY

This book is chock-full of stories because that's how we build relationships. Developing a relationship with you as a reader is very important to us. Through our stories, we dream of change. I've had my paradigm shift, and now we're dreaming of helping you make a shift or a change.

We're holding a vision of more people making exercise and self-care, including the exercise ball and active seating options, a fun part of every day. We want this book and CD-ROM to be used as a resource and a reference. We know this book gives you information that makes sense and has meaning. So take your time, digest it slowly, and revisit it often. We hope the ideas about exercise balls and active seating options, sensory baskets, and regulating your way through the day will help you find and maintain peace and balance in your life.

Finally, we wish you happy, healthy, active trails whether you are walking, running, biking, swimming, rolling, or bouncing along.

Appendix: Resources

www.anneontheball.com

For updates and information on the following information found in this book, check on this Web site:

- "Anne's Anchoring Ankrons" lap pads and neck weights for all ages
- Information on consultations for integrating the ideas from *Fitness on the Ball* into schools programs by Linda Kelly, Anne Spalding, and Anne Turnacliff
- Resources
- References
- Recommendations
- Workshop information for physical education
- Workshop information for classrooms
- Products related to active seating
- Products related to sensory basket items
- Sensory baskets
- Environmentally-friendly product suggestions, ideas, and availability

PRODUCTS AND COMPANIES

The following products and companies are mentioned in this book, and the companies can be contacted at the addresses, phone numbers, and Web sites listed with the product or company information.

Ball Dynamics International, LLC

14215 Mead Street
Longmont, CO 80504
1-800-752-2255
www.fitball.com

FitBALL: The Balanced Workout (DVD)

Designed by Joanne Posner-Mayer, P.T. and Lindsay Ross, this instructional video is perfect for post-rehab workouts. The *FitBALL The Balanced Workout* is a total-body routine for dynamic strengthening and joint and spinal mobility geared for the recovering patient.

Nontoxic Cleaner Recommendations

- Unbelievable! Green: Industrial Strength Cleaner & Degreaser
- Unbelievable! Citrus gel: Grease, Adhesives & Tar Remover

- www.coreproductsco.com
- Simple Green
- Tee Tree Oil- A few drops mixed in a spray bottle.

BOOKS

Ballinger, Eric. 1992. *The learning gym: Fun-to-do activities for success at school.* Ventura, CA: Edu-Kinesthetics. ISBN-13: 978-0942143096.

Dennison, Paul E., PhD, and Gail E. Dennison. 1989. *The edu-kinesthetics learning-through-movement series.* Ventura, CA: Edu-Kinesthetics. Revised edition, copyright 1994. Illustrations copyright 1988 by Gail E. Dennison.

- *Edu-K for Kids* (ISBN-13: 978-0942143010)
- *Brain Gym* (ISBN-13: 978-0942143058)
- *Brain Gym, Teacher's Edition* (ISBN-13: 978-0942143027)

Hallowell, E.M., and J.J. Ratey. 1995. *Driven to distraction.* New York, NY: Touchstone. ISBN-13: 978-0-684-80128-5

Hallowell, E.M., and J.J. Ratey. 1996. *Answers to distraction.* New York, NY: Bantam Books. ISBN-13: 978-0-553-37821-4

Kolberg, J. and K. Nadeau, PhD. 2002. *ADD-friendly ways to organize your life.* New York, NY: Routledge. ISBN 13: 978-1-58391-358-1

WEB SITE ARTICLES

Research samples of the use of exercise balls to improve focus and attention:

Attitude Magazine Editors. 2006. ADHD at school: Hyperactivity help strategies for harnessing ADHD hyperactivity in the classroom. *Attitude Magazine.* August/September 2006. Available: www.additudemag.com/adhd/article/1031.html.

Pytel, Barbara. 2007. No more classroom chairs. *Heron Marquez Estrada Star Tribune.* Oct. 27, 2007. Available: http://student-health-issues.suite101.com/article.cfm/no_more_classroom_chairs

Rynearson, P. 2008. Active classroom frees kids from desk chairs. *MSNBC.com.* March 28, 2006. Available: www.msnbc.msn.com/id/12055137/from/ET.

References

Bekoff, M. 2008. *Animals at play: Rules of the game.* Philadelphia: Temple University Press.

Bekoff, M., interview by Johanna Gallers, Dec. 24, 2008. How animal emotions parallel human lives: What animals can teach us about cooperation and compassion. KGNU Radio Metro. Boulder, CO.

Bevill, K. 2003. Gray Matters Brand Educational Cards. Littleton, CO: EnviroFriendly Printing.

Cranz, G. 2000. *The chair: Rethinking culture, body, and design.* New York: Norton.

Della Valle, J. 1984. An experimental investigation of the relationship(s) between preference for mobility and word recognition scores of seventh grade students to provide supervisory and administrative guidelines for the organization of effective instructional environments. Unpublished doctoral dissertation. New York: St. John's University.

Della Valle, J., et al. 1986. The effects of matching and mismatching students' mobility preferences on recognition and memory tasks. *Journal of Educational Research* 79(5): 267-72.

Doidge, N. 2007. *The brain that changes itself: Stories of personal triumph from the frontiers of brain science.* New York: Penguin Books.

Frick, S.M., R. Frick, P. Oetter, and E. Richter. 1996. *Out of the mouths of babes: Discovering the developmental significance of the mouth—A book especially for parents and other "grown-ups."* Hugo, MN: PDP Press.

Goleman, D. 1995. *Emotional intelligence: Why it can matter more than IQ.* New York: Bantam Books.

Hallowell, E.M., and J.J. Ratey. 1995. *Driven to distraction.* New York, NY: Touchstone.

———. 1996. *Answers to distraction.* New York, NY: Bantam Books.

Hannaford, C. 1995. *Smart moves: Why learning is not all in your head.* Arlington, VA: Great Ocean.

Healy, J.M. 2004. *Your child's growing mind.* New York: Broadway Books.

Holman, K. 2005. There is insufficient evidence (level 4) to support or refute the use of therapy balls as an alternative form of seating for improving classroom behaviour of children with autistic/behavioural disorders. Available: www.otcats.com/topics/CAT-kHolman2005.pdf.

Houston-Wilson, C., and L.J. Lieberman. 2002. *Strategies for inclusion: A handbook for physical educators.* Champaign, IL: Human Kinetics.

Illi, U. 1994. Balle statt stuhle im schulzimmer? (Balls instead of chairs in the classroom?). *Sporterzeihung in der schule,* June: 37-39.

Jensen, E. 1995. *The learning brain.* San Diego, CA: Turning Point.

———. 1996. *Brain-based learning.* Delmar, CA: Turning Point.

———. 2000. *Learning smarter: The new science of teaching.* Ed. Karen Markowitz. San Diego, CA: The Brain Store.

Kay, K., ed. 2000. *Uniquely gifted: Identifying and meeting the needs of the twice-exceptional student.* Gilsum, NH: Avocus Publishing.

Lamb, Wally. 2004. *Couldn't keep it to myself.* New York: HarperCollins.

O, the Oprah Magazine. 2009. Body wise: Posture power. February: 107.

Ratey, J.J. 2001. *A user's guide to the brain.* New York: Random House.

Ratey, J.J., with E. Hagerman. 2008. *Spark: The revolutionary new science of exercise and the brain.* New York: Little, Brown.

Rynearson, P. 2008. Active classroom frees kids from desk chairs. *MSNBC.com.* March 28, 2006. Available: www.msnbc.msn.com/id/12055137/from/ET.

Schwartz, J.M., and S. Begley. 2003. *The mind and the brain.* New York: HarperCollins.

Sousa, D.A. 2005. *How the brain learns to read.* Thousand Oaks, CA: Corwin Press.

———. 2006. *How the brain learns.* Thousand Oaks, CA: Corwin Press.

Spalding, A., L. Kelly, J. Santopietro, and J. Posner-Mayer. 1999. *Kids on the ball: Using Swiss balls in a complete fitness program.* Champaign, IL: Human Kinetics.

Virgilio, Stephen. 1997. *Fitness education for children: A team approach.* Champaign, IL: Human Kinetics.

Whiting, W.C., and R.F. Zernicke. 1998. *Biomechanics of musculoskeletal injury.* Champaign, IL: Human Kinetics.

Winfrey, O. 2009. What I know for sure. *O, the Oprah Magazine,* January: 190.

Glossary

abdominal muscles—Muscles of the lower front of the torso, including the rectus abdominis, obliquus abdominis externus, obliquus abdominis internus, and transverses abdominis.

active listener—A person who looks at the speaker, nods head to show they are attentive, and can paraphrase what the speaker said.

adductors—The adductor longus and the adductor magnus are muscles of the inner thigh that bring the legs together or across the midline.

aerobic exercise—Activity that improves the body's ability to use oxygen.

agonist muscle—The muscle moving the bones to which it is attached. Often called the prime mover. Depending on the movement, a muscle can be either an agonist or antagonist.

AIS—Active isolated stretching. A technique for stretching developed by Aaron Mattes. See www.stretchingusa.com.

antagonist muscle—The muscle whose action balances another associated muscle. The triceps is the antagonist of the biceps. The triceps relaxes when the biceps contracts and stabilizes the movement.

atrophy—The shrinking or gradual loss of tissue. Atrophy in a muscle is a loss of muscle mass.

balance—The ability of something or someone to maintain a steady position and not wobble or fall over.

base of support—The part or parts of the body that touch the floor (e.g., in walking, the base of support is the feet).

biceps femoris—One of the muscles in the back of the thigh; part of the hamstring muscle group.

biomechanics—The science that studies movement, posture, and body alignment and how it relates to mechanical principles.

brain—The control center of the central nervous system, responsible for behavior.

center of gravity—The center of an object's weight distribution where the force of gravity can be considered to act.

command center—Another term for the brain, emphasizing its importance in controlling our behavior.

control—A cue word to emphasize the student's mastery of his movement. Opposite of wild, careless, and thoughtless.

core strength—The strength of the muscles in the torso.

cortex—A portion of the brain that plays a key role in memory, attention, perceptual awareness, thought, language, and consciousness.

deltoid—A muscle of the shoulder that consists of three parts: anterior, lateral, and posterior.

dynamic balance—Balance while a person is moving, not stationary. It can be as simple as walking across the floor or as complex as walking on a balance beam.

elongate—To lengthen or make longer.

erector spinae—A group of muscles that extend from the sacrum, all along the vertebral column, along the length of the back.

exercise ball—Vinyl balls that can support up to 600 pounds (272 kg). Also called a stability ball, FitBall, physio-ball and Swiss ball.

fatigue zone—The point during exercise when muscles are tired and you start to slump in your workout.

Feldenkrais—A system of exercise for posture and bodily movement that builds focus and awareness of correct movement.

FITT—An acronym. F = frequency (how often per week), I = intensity (how hard), T = time (how long), and T = type (aerobic, strength, balance, flexibility).

flexibility—The ability of the joints in the body to move in a full range of motion. Developed by stretching.

frequency—The number of times per week someone completes a workout.

functional fitness—Fitness necessary to perform daily functions (e.g., to lift groceries, carry a toddler, or perform other daily tasks).

gastrocnemius—A muscle on the back part of the lower leg; also referred to as the calf.

gluteus—The gluteus consists of three parts (maximus, medius, and minimus) and comprises the buttocks.

gracilis—This muscle is located on the inside of the thigh and works along with the adductors to bring the leg toward the midline.

gravity—A force generated by the planet earth that exerts a pull on all objects and people toward the earth.

hamstrings—The hamstrings are located on the back of the thigh (upper leg). Consisting of the biceps femoris, semimembranosus, and semitendinosus, they act opposite to the quadriceps.

head—The part of the body that comprises the brain, eyes, ears, nose, and mouth.

hip flexors—A group of muscles that connect the femur (leg bone) and the pelvis and act to pull or bend the femur toward the torso.

hippocampus—The hippocampus is actually two parts of the forebrain and is located in the middle of the temporal lobes. It belongs to the limbic system and has a major role in short-term memory and spatial navigation.

intensity—Refers to how hard a person is working during exercise. Often measured by heart rate or perceived exertion.

latissimus dorsi—A pair of muscles on the lateral part (sides) of the back. They cover the lower part of the back and extend from the pelvic area to the armpit.

mindful—A cue word to emphasize that the learner is using her brain and thought process while moving.

muscle fibers—The cells that muscles are comprised of, which are called fibers because of their cylindrical shape.

neck—The part of the body that connects the head and shoulders.

nervous system—Refers to the brain, spinal cord, and nerves that form the connections for all messages from the brain and sensations to the brain.

neurobiology—The study of the nervous system's cells (soma) and the way these cells are organized into functional circuits that process information and modify or alter behavior (Schwartz 2003).

neurogenesis—The area that neurobiologists study, or the creation of new neural cells.

neuroplasticity—Changes in the brain as a result of experience, especially movement.

obliquus abdominis—Consists of the obliquus abdominis externus (the outermost and largest of the abdominal muscles), and the obliquus internus (which lies just underneath the external oblique). These muscles lie on the side of the trunk and work together to achieve torsional, or twisting, movement of the trunk.

off balance—Falling or wobbling. Unstable.

on balance—Not falling. Stable, whether stationary (static balance) or moving (dynamic balance).

overload—One of the principles of training. To improve a component of fitness, the muscle or system must work above its normal level.

pectineus—A muscle located on the inner side of the upper thigh. Its action is to assist in hip flexion and adduction.

pectoralis major—The large muscles of the upper chest. They cover the chest from the sternum to the armpit.

physical activity—The body moving. Includes house and yard work as well as sport and fitness activities.

Pilates—A system of exercise developed by Joseph Pilates. Includes exercises that focus on the body's core.

piriformis—A small muscle that lies under the gluteus muscles and connects between the sacrum and the femur.

posture—Refers to the alignment of the body when standing or sitting.

progression—A principle of training. To improve a fitness component, exercise must gradually get more difficult by increasing the frequency, intensity, or duration (time).

prone—Front of the body on or toward the floor (belly down).

proper mechanics—The optimal posture or body positioning and alignment used when performing an exercise or skill.

proprioceptors—Sensors in the limbs that provide information about joint angle, muscle length, and tension.

quadriceps—The four large muscles on the front of the upper leg (rectus femoris, vastus lateralis, vastus medialis, and vastus intermedius).

regression—A principle of training. A muscle or bodily system will return to it previous state if exercise is not done on a regular basis.

repetition—A term used in fitness training to indicate the number of times an exercise is performed before resting. Usually referred to as *reps*.

resistance—To work against. In building muscle strength, resistance is provided by weights, tubing, bands and other pieces of equipment. The lifting, lowering, pushing, and pulling of these objects is work the muscle does to overcome the resistance.

sartorius—Muscle on the upper front of the leg. It acts to rotate the femur internally and flex the knee.

scapulae—A pair of bones located on the upper back and often called the shoulder blades. Triangular in shape, they connect the humerus (arm bone) with the clavicle (collar bone) and form the shoulder girdle.

sensory baskets—The concept of regulatory items and equipment to give suggestions and choices to teachers and students about how to regulate their way through the day.

sensory integration—The ability to integrate or bring together all the information that comes to us through our senses (seeing, hearing, smelling, tasting, and feeling).

serratus anterior—A muscle connecting the upper eight ribs and the scapulae. The two serratus anterior muscles help stabilize the scapulae and play a major role in posture.

set—A term used in exercise to indicate a certain group of repetitions (e.g., "Perform two sets of 10 repetitions").

skull—The bony portion of the head. The skull supports the facial features and protects the brain.

soleus—A muscle in the back of the lower leg; along with the gastrocnemius, it is called the calf.

specificity—In fitness, specificity is a concept that only one aspect of a component can be addressed at a time. For example, cardiorespiratory activity, like running, develops endurance; however it will not develop flexibility. In the same manner, working the legs in a strength workout will not improve arm strength.

spinal cord—The bundle of nerves that go from the brain through the vertebrae of the back to the pelvis.

static balance—In balancing, static means in place, not moving.

static stretch—A stretch that is held motionless. No bouncing.

steady—In balancing, steady refers to not swaying, not wobbling, and not falling.

strength—The ability of muscles to exert force. Muscles can lift, lower, push, pull, hold, and press.

supine—Back of the body close to or on the floor (belly up).

tai chi—An exercise form originating in China that uses slow-motion movements.

time—Refers to how long a person spends doing a particular exercise.

torso—The trunk of the body, extending from the neck to the pelvis, excluding the limbs.

trapezius—The large superficial muscle of the upper back that moves both the neck and shoulders.

triceps—A muscle of the upper arm on the back side, opposite the biceps.

vertebrae—The bony portion of the skeleton that forms the spine.

weight transfer—Shifting of body weight from one body part to another. Can be achieved by steplike movements, rocking, or rolling.

wobbly—Not stable. Moving back and forth over the balance point and appearing as if you are about to fall.

yoga—System of exercises involving poses that develop flexibility, balance, and strength.

About the Authors

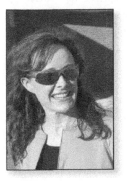

Anne Spalding is an elementary physical education teacher in Boulder, Colorado. Throughout the years she's presented physical education curricula at state, district, and national conventions with her friend and mentor, Anne Turnacliff, and coauthor, Linda Kelly. Promoting the value of exercise balls has been an integral part of many of her presentations.

In 1997 she received the Torch of Hope award from the American Heart Association, and in 1999 she was named the Colorado Physical Education Teacher of the Year. She is a member of the American Alliance for Health, Physical Education, Recreation and Dance as well as the Colorado Alliance for Health, Physical Education, Recreation and Dance.

Anne has worked on and received grant awards for community health education, integration, and innovations. In Adams County District 12 she was a part of the Voices Against Violence grant. She is currently cochair of the Crest View Elementary Peer Mediation and Conflict Resolution program. Promoting peer mediation is an important aspect of Anne's teaching. She and her students have witnessed the benefits of kids talking to kids to resolve conflict and to enhance communication skills.

Near and dear to Anne's heart is studying Spanish. This lifetime adventure has broadened her cultural and linguistic skills. Anne also enjoys biking, hiking, camping, skiing, snowshoeing, and spending time with her family and friends.

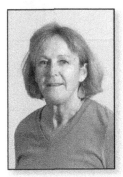

Linda Kelly, EdD, is a retired physical education teacher who lives in Longmont, Colorado. She taught elementary physical education in Boulder Valley Schools for over 30 years and was an adjunct professor at Colorado University for six years. She taught a course for future classroom teachers that emphasized the importance of physical activity and included experiential lessons on ways that movement can be incorporated into the classroom (including active seating).

During her teaching career, Linda's focus was motor learning, physical activity, and fitness. She was awarded numerous grants for heart health promotion, physical activity, and fitness, all in an effort to enrich the physical education experience of her students. Linda shared her programs at district in-services, state conventions (CAAHPERD), district conventions (Central District), and national conventions (AAHPERD). She presented on volleyball, homemade equipment, New Games, challenge activities, and exercise ball activities as well as heart monitors and pedometers.

Linda has published two articles in the *Physical Education Newsletter* and a research article in *Pediatric Exercise Science*. She also coauthored *Kids on the Ball* with Anne Spalding. Linda earned her MA in physical education with a focus on motor learning from the University of California at Santa Barbara. She earned her doctorate in physical education pedagogy from the University of Northern Colorado.

Linda's interest in using exercise balls began in 1990 when she met Joanne Posner Mayer at a CAHPERD convention. Since then she has taught with the balls. Her students have included kindergartners through sixth-graders and senior adults. Linda also facilitated the use of active seating in the classrooms at her elementary school.

Currently her interests are personal fitness (exercise ball workouts, hiking, walking, and lifting weights), qi gong, gardening, writing, reading, and spending time with her adult children. She also is addicted to Sudoku and has started solving crossword puzzles.

SYSTEM REQUIREMENTS

You can use this CD-ROM on either a Windows-based PC or a Macintosh computer.

Windows

- IBM PC compatible with Pentium processor
- Windows 98/2000/XP/Vista
- Adobe Reader 8.0
- 4x CD-ROM drive

Macintosh

- Power Mac recommended
- System 10.4 or higher
- Adobe Reader
- 4x CD-ROM drive

USER INSTRUCTIONS

Windows

1. Insert the *Fitness on the Ball* CD-ROM. (Note: The CD-ROM must be present in the drive at all times.)
2. Select the "My Computer" icon from the desktop.
3. Select the CD-ROM drive.
4. Open the file you wish to view. See the "00Start.pdf" file for a list of the contents.

Macintosh

1. Insert the *Fitness on the Ball* CD-ROM. (Note: The CD-ROM must be present in the drive at all times.)
2. Double-click the CD icon located on the desktop.
3. Open the file you wish to view. See the "00Start" file for a list of the contents.

For customer support, contact Technical Support:
Phone: 217-351-5076 Monday through Friday (excluding holidays) between 7:00 a.m. and 7:00 p.m. (CST).
Fax: 217-351-2674
E-mail: support@hkusa.com

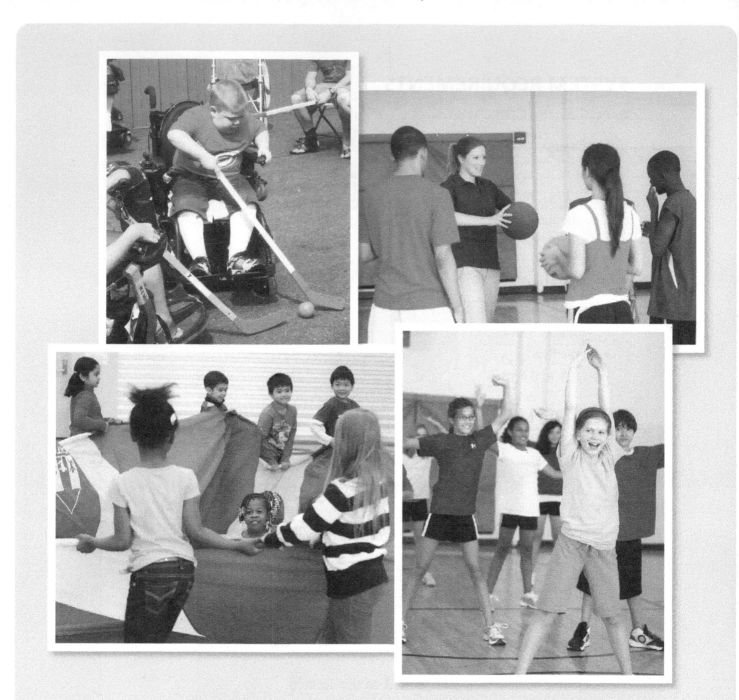

You'll find other outstanding
physical education resources at

www.HumanKinetics.com